Peter Downey became an author because all the eighties rock-star jobs were taken. He lives in the suburbs with his wife, three children and a minivan he's owned for twenty years. Peter is the best-selling author of several books on parenting, marriage and religious topics; he has written for a range of journals and magazines and at various times has had his face on television and his voice on radio discussing all things parental.

With Bachelor, Masters and Doctoral degrees in education, arts and leadership, Peter's mild-mannered alter ego is an English teacher and Deputy Principal at an independent school in Sydney, Australia. So if you email him, make sure you use correct grammar and punctuation.

Peter wrote this book because he believes somebody should warn dads-to-be about the enormous changes fatherhood will bring to their lives. He wrote this book because he believes that dads are important and, in short, children need good dads. He wrote this book to let anxious and unprepared not-yet-dads know that being a dad is great and that everything will be okay in the end. However, he mostly wrote this book so he could become famous and retire to a villa in Portugal.

You can contact Peter at author@peterdowney.com.au
and visit www.peterdowney.com.au
or www.facebook.com/peterdowneyauthor.au

Also by Peter Downey

So You're Going to Be a Dad
Dads, Toddlers and the Chicken Dance
Everything a Bloke Needs to Know About Marriage
Inspired Stuff: Everything you wanted to know about the
Bible but were afraid to ask
(with Ben Shaw)

SO YOU'RE GOING TO BE A
DAD

REVISED EDITION

Peter Downey

Da Capo
LIFE
LONG

A Member of the Perseus Books Group

North American revised edition copyright © Da Capo Press 2016
Text © Peter Downey 2014
Illustrations © Nik Scott 1994

Typeset by Midland Typesetters, Australia

First published in Australia in 2014 as SO YOU'RE GOING TO BE A DAD 20-YEAR ANNIVERSARY EDITION by
Simon & Schuster (Australia) Pty Limited
Suite 19A, Level 1, 450 Miller Street, Cammeray, NSW 2062
Original and revised editions published by Simon & Schuster Australia 1994, 2005

Library of Congress Cataloging-in-Publication Data

Names: Downey, Peter.
Title: So you're going to be a dad / Peter Downey.
Other titles: So you are going to be a dad
Description: Revised Da Capo Press edition. | Boston, MA : Da Capo Lifelong, a member of the Perseus Books Group, 2016. | Includes bibliographical references and index.
Identifiers: LCCN 2015044940| ISBN 9780738219066 (paperback) | ISBN 9780738219073 (e-book)
Subjects: LCSH: Fatherhood. | BISAC: FAMILY & RELATIONSHIPS / Parenting / Fatherhood. | HEALTH & FITNESS / Pregnancy & Childbirth. | HUMOR / Topic / Marriage & Family.
Classification: LCC HQ756 .D59

Revised Da Capo Press edition 2016
Published by Da Capo Press
A Member of the Perseus Books Group
www.dacapopress.com

Da Capo Press books are available at special discounts for bulk purchases in the U.S. by corporations, institutions, and other organizations. For more information, please contact the Special Markets Department at the Perseus Books Group, 2300 Chestnut Street, Suite 200, Philadelphia, PA, 19103, or call (800) 810-4145, ext. 5000, or e-mail special.markets@perseusbooks.com.

10 9 8 7 6 5 4 3 2 1

This book is dedicated to my children,
Rachael, Georgia and Matilda,
whom I ignored for six months
while I wrote a book on how to be a good dad

Contents

Author's Note

"You know . . . when I was nineteen, Grandpa took me
on the roller-coaster . . . up . . . down . . . up . . . down . . .
Oh, what a ride! Some didn't like it. They went on the
merry-go-round. That just goes around . . . nothing.
I like the roller-coaster. You get more out of it."
Helen Shaw (Grandma), *Parenthood*

So, you're going to be a dad?

Well, from one dad to another, here's a couple of tips
you might find useful.

First, in the last trimester of your wife's pregnancy, hire
a pager so that, whenever she goes into labor, she can buzz
you straight away, no matter where you are. And, second,
have a bag of quarters in your car at all times. That way, once
your child is born, you can use the payphone in the hospital
lobby to call your immediate family and friends with the
good news.

Awesome advice . . . *right?*

Um . . . well . . . maybe not so much *now*. But it wasn't that long ago that mobile phones were still the ridiculously brick-like and expensive toys of only the rich and famous, and pagers and coins were de rigueur for the impending father. Which is why I wrote about them when this book first came out.

But here we are, twenty years later, and things have changed.

(If this book were a movie, this is where it would suddenly go *flashback*, using techniques such as a swirling screen, change to black and white, and a dramatically descending scale run down a xylophone . . . so let's go back . . . *back* . . . *back* . . .)

As a soon-to-be-dad, it would be an understatement to suggest that when I found out my wife, Meredith, was pregnant with our first child I was anything short of terrified . . . with that special kind of terror only known to clueless new dads and rabbits caught in headlights on a country road.

As a way of processing the whole magnitude of impending fatherhood, I suppose, I started a journal detailing my thoughts, feelings and experiences. It began as a kind of diary written to no one in particular, documenting our journey as we navigated the unknown turf of pregnancy, childbirth and eventually parenthood. And writing seemed a more constructive use of my time than rocking back 'n' forth in a dark corner mumbling, "But I don't want to change diapers . . ."

Pretty soon, that little journal grew into a stack of pages of anecdotes, facts, random thoughts, curious discoveries, quirky stories, personal asides and hitherto unknown minutiae from the world of new parenting. Several of my friends – fellow dads-to-be – started borrowing what I grandiosely referred to as "my book," and asking for more. And so it was that, almost on a whim, I old-school printed a copy and posted it to a publisher and . . . without wanting to sound too flippant . . . the rest, as they say, is history.

My publisher printed my ramblings – now with its own whimsically rhetorical title, *So You're Going to Be a Dad* – and the first print run sold well. It was soon reprinted, and then reprinted, and then, after another reprint, it got reprinted again. And again. I lost track after a while. It began selling in New Zealand, Canada, the United Kingdom and, inexplicably, places such as Turkey, Korea and Nepal. I even had to translate a special edition for American release (because in Australia, babies wear nappies, not "diapers.")

Along with the book came radio interviews, TV spots, and magazine and newspaper articles. The ABC's *Australian Story* spent a week following us around for an episode about me as "the reluctant dad." The front page of *The Sydney Morning Herald* dubbed the book "barbecue wisdom"; the kind of homespun chat that a bunch of guys might have around a sizzling hotplate of T-bones while they offered each other engineering advice about the intricacies of travel-crib assembly. On several occasions, I was even referred to as a "parenting expert," which my own children find both hilarious and ridiculous.

The most unexpected thing was the number of emails I received from guys (and, surprisingly, from their partners) from New Zealand to Nepal and lots of other places that don't even start with "N" to say *g'day and thanks* for the book. They connected with the clueless author and were somehow reassured to discover that they were not the only new parent on the planet trying to work out their mixed feelings of inadequacy and joy about being a dad (or mom). I am flattered that this book seems to have comforted and amused many people in the face of parenthood.

But parenting stuff changes over time. Every generation's experience of pregnancy, birth and parenting is a reflection of the customs, practices and attitudes of their time, which are in turn affected by changing technologies, laws, community norms, discoveries, inventions and expectations. And it's been that way since before my Great Aunty Dot was sent galloping across the fields on Bessie, the old grey nag, to fetch Doc Williamson from town and bring him back quickly, girl, for Winnie's water has done and broke. *Boil the water! Tear the sheets!*

In the twenty years since *So You're Going to Be a Dad* first hit the shelves and I was elbow deep in diapers, much has changed. The internet now provides a wealth of information about parenting that was previously not available; ultrasounds have gone high-tech; advice on preventing sudden infant death syndrome has done a 360, and then a 180; there are more baby gadgets and gizmos on the market than ever before; government legislation around matters such as paid parental leave, Caesarean births and home births have impacted common practices; digital technologies and social media have totally redefined the way new parents record and share the whole shebang (#annoyingstatusupdating); to say nothing of the rise of those bastards who run down narrow sidewalks with jogger strollers, scattering pedestrians like bowling pins.

So, twenty years later, it's time for an update and spruce up, and this Revised Edition is it. (Think of it like the Special Edition re-release of the *Star Wars* films, but without that stupid bit at the end of Episode VI where old ghost Anakin was replaced by young ghost Anakin.)

A lot has changed over that time in my own life too. The words in this book paint a picture of a world far removed from the one in which I now live. My three daughters are now eating solid foods and are out of diapers. Which is a good thing, because they're all in college. (Yes, amazingly and unpredictably, they are all still alive and relatively well-adjusted individuals, giving hope to hapless dads the world over.) So rereading the original book for me is like leafing through an old photo album full of pictures I can barely remember ... Oh well, that's what happens, I suppose. Time flies, kids grow up and I wear my trousers rolled. Literally. (Your time will come.)

But while the frills and trappings around parenting continue to change, some things are timeless, and the core of this book remains the same. It still takes a sperm and ovum to create life. A woman still bears a baby for nine months, after which, one way or another, it has to come out. And then the baby comes home ... and life is never the same again. The relationship a dad has with his son or daughter is critical. You are important, now more than ever in this internet age where there are competing forces trying to "raise" your kids, not all of them worthy. Because know this: if you don't raise your child, someone or something else will.

As I read over the First Edition of the book – which remains the core of this Revised Edition – I sometimes fear that as a new dad I appear too flippant, too negative, too scared, too incompetent, too stupid, too self-centered and too ignorant. *Was I really like that?* Well ... yeah, I suspect I was. In revising this book, the temptation has been to change that tone, to reinvent and rewrite myself as a new dad who was confident, learned, positive, loving, capable, eager and basically less of a complainer and a whiner than the bozo you read about here. As the dad of three young women now, having emerged from the other side of the parenting tunnel, I want to grab my young-dad self by the collar, give me a good slap and say, "Get over it and get on with it. It's not *that* hard. What's the big deal, you whiner?" But that wouldn't be right. I don't want to discount those very real feelings and experiences I had as a clueless guy in my mid-twenties just because I can't remember them now. It's too easy to reinterpret the past. And it would be disingenuous to do so. So I have left my neurotic and inept self untouched. I hope you can relate to him . . . I mean . . . um, me.

The original cover illustration of this book depicted a naive new dad looking up at a signpost indicating two destinations. One destination reads "Having a Life," while the other, pointing in the opposite direction, says "Being a Dad." That rather pessimistic and bleak interpretation of things made perfect sense to me when Meredith was first pregnant and I had no idea what was ahead. The naive soon-to-be dad was me, contemplating the future. "Life" and "Dad" seemed mutually exclusive. The *old* was going. A *new* was coming.

And . . . that turned out to be exactly right. One hundred percent. Life as I knew it ended with my wife's pregnancy. What I wasn't prepared for, however, was that that turned out to be just fine. Life became infinitely and indescribably better. From shaky and hesitant beginnings, being a husband and dad has been the best and most important and most enjoyable thing I have done in my life. It has redefined me and everything in my world. Maybe that sounds scary and weird from where you are right now, sitting reading this book and staring down the dark tunnel of impending fatherhood. But trust me . . . on the other side of the tunnel, the sun is shining, the grass is green and the water is fine.

So let's go back to the beginning, a very good place to start . . . because your wife is pregnant and, at some point soon . . . you're going to be a dad.

Disclaimers

Just before you *do* start wading through this book in earnest, there are . . . ahem . . . a handful of things I'd like to bring to your attention:

1. What you are about to read is born out of my own experiences, knowledge and opinions. It is a general book, reflecting Meredith's and my journey through a garden variety suburban pregnancy, hospital childbirth and red-brick-in-the-suburbs parenting situation. Keep in mind that every pregnancy is different. No labor is the same. Each baby is unique. Doctors' views differ. People have varied attitudes and opinions. Practices and technologies evolve. Hospitals have different facilities. Policies change. Averages are just that – averages. So, whatever you do, don't read this book as though it's a join-the-dots Sinai-delivered parenting User's Manual.

2. Some of the things I touch on here in a casual aside are the topics of their own weighty tomes. I have erred on the side of simplicity and brevity, and have avoided specialist matters that require great sensitivity or academic consideration. You will not find in this book any lengthy and tangential explorations of, for example, IVF, miscarriage, home birth, umbilical-cord clamping, the particular issues posed by twins and triplets, attachment parenting or alternative medicines.

3. In talking about the female person who will form the other half of the parenting team in your family, I have used the word

"wife" instead of "partner." Sure, not everyone who becomes a dad or mom is married, but, according to the National Center for Health Statistics, two-thirds of births are "in marriage," so "wife" it is. And, in referring to the baby in the book, I have called it either "the baby" or "it." I know it sounds impersonal and objectifying, but I just couldn't make up my mind. And it's my book, so I can do anything I damn well like.

4. The internet has massively altered the experience of the soon-to-be-dad – in terms of access to information, support, social connection and so on. There are thousands of great websites and blogs that would be good for you to check out. But in this book I have avoided listing them because, in short, I don't know if they'll be there tomorrow.

5. Finally, I acknowledge that this book is not everyone's cup of java. There's the odd nasty review floating around the internet – and man, I do mean *na-a-asty* – and a group of American birth assistants took out a fatwa on me, claiming this book disrespects and degrades the beauty of pregnancy and the awe and spiritual wonderment of birth. In addition, lots of people are quite opinionated and passionate (#psycho) about what's what when it comes to pregnancy and birth and parenting: websites, blogs and online forums go into battle over circumcision, immunization, breast v. bottle feeding and even cloth v. disposable diapers, and if you don't agree with them . . . then you are the spawn of Satan and your child is going to leave home at twelve and end up on crystal meth. I hope you like my approach, but, if not, I am but one voice among many in the wealth of new-parent writing out there.

Peter Downey
2014

Prologue

Being a dad has its advantages and disadvantages.

Advantages
- A decade, guaranteed, of guilt-free Disney/Pixar animated movies on the big screen.
- Rediscovering your love of Lego.
- Social kudos in your workplace, especially among women.
- People usher you to the front of lines.
- You can break wind anytime, anyplace and blame it on the baby.
- The joyous fulfillment of playing a significant part in the life of another human being.

Disadvantages
- Life, as you know it, is over.

This is a book about being a dad. I wrote it for three reasons.

First, I wanted to become the rich and famous author of a book with one of those "Three Million Now in Print" stickers on it. (That didn't exactly come to fruition. However, I have sold over a hundred thousand copies, and with the publishing royalties I have been able to put a full set of new tires on my minivan. On at least three separate occasions. Yay.)

Second, I'm writing this book to warn you. Becoming a dad is life-changing. Monumentally, teeth-crackingly, awe-inspiringly life-changing. Somebody needs to tell you. It might as well be me.

My wife, Meredith, and I are the proud parents of three daughters: Rachael, Georgia and Matilda. And I do mean proud. I love my kids. I love being their dad.

Except for that time Rachael redecorated her room by pulling the cap off a container of baby powder.

And except for that time when, during a dinner party, Georgia appeared pants-less and clutching a nuggety shape, causing one of our dinner guests to ask, incorrectly, "Where'd ya get that pine cone, Georgie?"

And especially except for that time Tilly ran through a plate-glass door wearing only silky pajamas, sending us scurrying to the hospital in one of those "Please God" moments.

Yep, there's nothing quite like being a dad. I consider myself a fully fledged family man. Being a dad is really important to me. It is at the very core of who I am. But it was a bit of a rocky beginning and I certainly wouldn't claim to have enjoyed every minute of it. As a new dad, I remember crawling into bed each night mumbling inanely to myself, *Why didn't anybody tell me about this? Why wasn't I warned? Can I change my mind about this whole dad thing?*

I remember feeling angry that I had subscribed to an ideal that being a dad was easy and fun and full of warmth and wonder and soft-focus, TV-commercial moments made up of throwing a ball in the park and cooking burgers around a campfire in the backyard. I felt miffed that the brotherhood-of-guys had failed to adequately and truthfully prepare me for my new station in life. Then again . . . it wouldn't be the first time the brotherhood-of-guys has let me down and been misleading. It is they, after all, who also suggest that paintball doesn't hurt, that getting a stripper is a good way to finish a bachelor party or that getting a fully sick Chinese character tatt on your bicep while on holiday in Phuket is a good idea.

Becoming a dad is a shock to the system. It's not like getting a new car or wide-screen TV. So I'm writing to give you the lowdown, the scoop, the big picture, the rope-a-dope, the man-in-the-street, guy-next-door view.

Third, I have a strong conviction about the importance of dadhood. Our country needs good dads. Our kids need good dads. They need their dads to love them, care for them, know them, teach them, raise them, spend time with them, discipline them, throw them up in the air and wrestle them on the carpet.

It makes me happy that lots of men take an active and involved role in family life. Unfortunately, some guys still view parenting as a maternal thing. They see their role as bread-winner and beer-drinker. This is a tragedy. As far as I can ascertain, there are only five parenting things that men can't do:

- get pregnant
- carry a baby for nine months

- give birth
- breastfeed
- remember the names of all the kids at playgroup.

As a culture, we still tend to define ourselves by the work we do, and that can lead some men to get the balance wrong. I have met dads who are not into family stuff, dads who seem permanently away on business, dads who are perpetually busy and are so wrapped up in their own lives that they and their children only ever pass like ships in the night. They are men with no time for family.

I was leafing through a stack of old magazines the other day when I came across an article on the new breed of workaholics: men who seem to live for their work and have little or no time for their own kids. It's my belief that, one day, these men will wake up and look at their children who don't know them . . . and realize too late that there is more to life than work.

So, in writing this book, I hope that I help some guys – maybe you? – realize how important and how enjoyable (albeit sometimes frustrating) it is to be "Dad."

But how exactly do you "be a dad"?

Good question. Unfortunately, us guys can't go to night school to get a certification in Fathering and, as far as I know, universities don't offer Bachelor degrees in Paternity. How do we, as aspiring fathers-to-be, learn the ropes of fathering without hanging ourselves, so to speak? When Meredith was pregnant with our first child, Rachael, I had a thousand questions that needed answering. There were plans to be made and things to do, and I knew nothing about babies and parenting and kids. And I do mean *nothing*. I needed information and advice to help me work out, essentially, *what is it exactly that I'm supposed to do?*

I started looking for decent books that would prepare me for parenting. You can spot these books by their promising titles, such as *The Complete Guide to Parenting . . .* or *How to Raise a Child . . .* or *Ten Easy Steps to . . .* Either that or by their covers, which feature soft-focus photos of models (with pregnancy-suggesting cushions stuffed up their cashmere cardigans) silhouetted in frosted bay windows staring out to the middle distance with a serene look on their face that says, "I'm pregnant and I'm in love with my baby . . ."

I have to say, I didn't find too many books that really did the trick. Most are written for women, many adopting a kind of alternate-reality saccharine insipidness to which I could not relate. The few dad books I stumbled across (squeezed in among other non-male books such as *Your Breast, Your Baby* or *Terrifically Trim After Childbirth*) were sort of okay but tended to be either dry and technical textbooks (which put me to sleep) or clichéd dad collages with inspirational desktop-calendar quotations (which were cute – "A father carries photos where his money used to be" – but didn't actually tell me anything).

Somewhere in there, I decided to write this.

Which raises the question: who exactly is Peter Downey to be telling me about all this stuff anyway?

Well, I'm not a child psychologist, bioethicist, obstetrician or pediatrician. I'm not the head of some amazing parent-education organization. And although I'm a "Doctor," my Doctorate is in education not medicine, which means I am perpetually anxious that on a long-haul flight an attendant will call out, "Is anyone here a doctor?" and I'll put up my hand but, despite my attempts to qualify that statement, I'll be whisked to the back of the plane, there to conduct a Caesarean with nothing but airline cutlery and a plastic sewing kit, and afterwards we'll all have a good old laugh about the misunderstanding.

My main qualification is that I'm an ordinary guy, husband and dad of three kids. I live in the suburbs, work five days a week, wash the car on the weekend and like to watch movies and get Thai takeout on a Friday night.

One day, I was a normal, carefree guy, just like you. The next day, I was buying diapers and trying to assemble a travel crib. If anything, it is my inadequacies and failings, not my expertise, that make this book what it is. So here I am, a few years down the track, ready to share my joys, frustrations, ideas and mistakes. If that doesn't convince you, though, I've watched plenty of films and TV shows with dads and babies in them.

The basic message of this book is that being a dad takes energy, commitment and involvement. It takes a lot of time and effort. You can't do it half-heartedly. You can't do it in your spare time. This is very important for you to understand, so I'm going to write it again.

Being a dad takes energy, commitment and involvement. It takes a lot of time and effort. You can't do it half-heartedly. You can't do it in your spare time.

It means being active and involved in the daily dealings with your baby. It means "getting your hands dirty" – metaphorically and literally – and participating in all aspects of family life. It means sharing the parenting and rejecting outdated stereotypes that parenting is "women's business." If you haven't got the point yet, read this paragraph again.

Our kids need us. Your baby, whether you've met it yet or not, needs you. It needs your testosterone, your love, care, concern, involvement, wisdom, strength, patience and discipline. It needs your strong arm and your gentle hand. It needs you to be there, to be involved, and you've got to know them, know when to hold them, and know when to fold them . . . hang on a sec . . .

Obviously, this book is primarily intended for soon-to-be or new dads, the man who knows little or nothing about fatherhood but who wants to face the storm and be the best damn dad he can be. But the absence of discussion here around moms or particular maternal issues should in no way lessen the obvious importance of moms or detract from the integral relationship of the husband–wife parenting team. Moms are as equally important as dads. I have nothing against women. In fact, I like women.

I even married one.

So welcome to the wonderful world of fatherhood. We have a long road ahead of us. A hard road. A road fraught with obstacles, trials and tribulations. But it is also a rewarding road, adorned with great experiences and golden moments that you wouldn't have thought possible. And once you walk the road, you'll never be the same again.

So, good luck on your journey.

You'll need it.

1

And So, It Begins

"If only I could have seen the writing on the wall. It would have said, 'Your wife's pregnant! Run away! Run away!'"

Sex and its Side Effects

WARNING: The Surgeon General advises that sex may cause children.

Sex is an appropriate starting point for our consideration of fatherhood. After all, this is where the journey begins.

By the very virtue of the fact that you are actually reading this page, let's assume that you have already passed this initial but crucial test. With flying colors. In the interests of good taste, I shall therefore refrain from elaborating any further on how much fun you had in the process and "Was it good for you too, babe?," etc.

But we all get the message. While you were lying back in a haze of post-coital euphoria – like they do in the movies – an armada of about 300 million of your sperms set off from Port Penis on the first leg of their marathon swim through all that female plumbing, the names of which I can never quite remember.

(I will probably never come to terms with all those bits and pieces of the female anatomy. As a teenager, sitting in a Personal Development class at an all-boys' school, I was always perplexed by the textbook cross-sections of women's insides. You know the picture I mean? Yeah, the diagram of the one-legged woman. I could never follow all the bulbous squiggles and wormy channels with the funny names. In fact, it was only years later that I discovered that the cross-section diagram was in fact a *side* view, not a *top* view. (A tip: the *top* view looks like a Rorschach ink blot of a bat spreading its wings.) Maybe I should have paid more attention, instead of sitting at the back of the classroom with Adam Armstrong trying to put sample diaphragms on our heads like swimming caps.)

Anyway, while nothing to you, those several centimeters from the tip of the penis to their intended destination are an Olympic endurance event to these little tadpoles. They will only survive for a few days, so there is no time to waste. Like salmon battling upstream, they have to swim from the vagina, north through the uterus (or womb), and climb up one of the two Fallopian tubes to where an egg (more correctly an ovum, or the less well-known oocyte) is hiding, or soon to arrive.

Now, let's just pause to reflect for a moment on what's happening here. Before your child is even close to being *created*, this is already an amazing feat. To transpose it into human terms and dimensions, think of it like this. Imagine

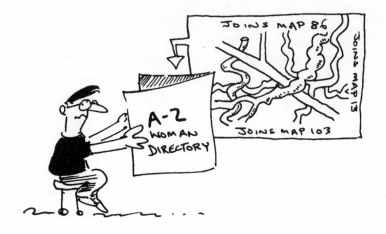

you (representing a sperm) are competing in a biathlon. You and the entire population of Brazil (all the other sperms) are shot down a three-mile urethral chute at around fifteen times the speed of sound. You splash down into an unpleasantly acidic subterranean ocean, in total darkness, and have to locate and swim for a half-mile through a secret tunnel that is only fifty or so yards wide, before emerging into, well, let's say Long Island Sound. And then the race is really on. You've still got three miles left, still in total darkness.

Swimmers around you are dying by the tens of millions, just exhausted, or victims of aggressive antibodies, or swimming off somewhere lost and never to be seen again. It's chaos. A couple of hours later, there are only a few thousand competitors left.

At the far end of the sound, there are two tributaries heading off in opposite directions, and you have to decide which one to swim up. It's a big choice. Only one of them will contain the treasured prize – an ovum, which to you is an orb about the size of a double-decker bus – and, even then, only if your timing is just right and you happen to arrive at that exact moment each month when it happens to pass by.

And so you and the last remaining few hundred of the strongest swimmers head off, desperately hoping that it's all been worthwhile . . . (It's amazing when you think about it that humans exist at all.)

Post-intercourse, while you are going about your ordinary life (making breakfast or snoring or heading back to work after your "lunchbreak"), you and your wife are both probably blissfully oblivious to all this mysterious and wonderful action taking place inside her body on a microscopic level. And the ovum hasn't even appeared yet!

The ovum is the smallest cell in the human body that can be seen with the naked eye . . . although I can't really imagine a situation where this would come to pass. Being about the width of a human hair, it makes the period at the end of this sentence look like a beach ball. The point is that it is very, very small.

The ovum has undergone a journey of its own. Women have about half a million of these ova stored in their ovaries. Each month during ovulation, a mature or "ripe" ovum leaves its sisters and bobs on down one of the Fallopian tubes, like a little planet wondering if the strange aliens with the tails will perhaps come and visit.

It's a pretty narrow window and time is critical, because this ovum has a "use-by" date of only about twenty-four hours. Either it arrives and waits to see if any sperms turn up, or the sperms are already there, hanging around impatiently. They could have been there for a few days already, although after seventy-two hours they are really running out of steam for the second stage of the biathlon.

By now, there aren't too many sperms left. (One book I read described it as "a handful of sperm," a mental picture that I could have done without.) To return to our human-scale analogy, out of the original field of a few hundred million, it's now down to you and the final fifty swimmers, now surrounding the bus-sized orb, desperately trying to get inside first. Because that's the point. There is only one winner. Only one prize. First one in wins. The rest just swim off and die.

The sperms all find a spot on the ovum they can call their own, stick their heads down and start spinning around and around like fence-post diggers. Picture a tennis ball swarming with animated alfalfa sprouts. The winner is the first one to break the ovum wall and get in.

Two things immediately happen. The tail breaks off from the head of the successful sperm and the ovum gets coy and undergoes a chemical change, which instantly shuts out all the other contenders. It's a bit of a disappointment for them, I should imagine: getting all that way, beating all those odds, only to be defeated in the last second.

Sad, really.

Anyway, at that specific moment, what you have there is your child. Sure, it's only a single cell, technically and unromantically referred to as a zygote, but your child nonetheless, sitting in its own little dark, warm universe. You can almost imagine the Starship Enterprise zooming past through this microscopic universe with Spock at the view-screen musing, "It's life, Jim, but not as we know it."

And there you have it. The wheels of fate have spun in their diurnal course and, although you don't know it yet, the rest of your life has just massively changed direction. In short, you're going to be a dad.

This is the miracle of life. The miracle of sex. And it *is* a miracle.

God really was very clever to have thought it up.

This child of yours is unique in the universe. You and your wife are the only combination in history who could have created it. Think of it this way: your wife has about half a million ova. You have about 300 million sperms per ejaculation. Let us assume, for the sake of argument and mathematical convenience, that you have sex once a week over a ten-year potential parenting period. Your child could be *any combination* of any single sperm and any single ovum. So, if my mathematics serves me correctly (which it might not do, considering my grades at school), then that makes your child one of 78,000,000,000,000,000 (seventy-eight quadrillion) possible people combinations.

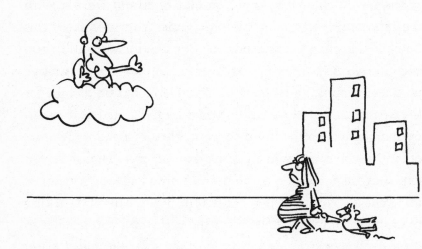

This is a humbling thing for a father to contemplate. Without getting into a philosophical debate, it's kind of awesome to think about the incredibly complex and infinitesimal beginnings of human life – the beginnings of the life of your child. What is at this point an indistinct speck will grow to be a person whom you will know and love intimately – a person, I might add, who will change your life and take you into a world you could not have possibly imagined.

You will see this infinitesimally small spot learn to crawl, walk and talk. It will keep you up at night. You will spend countless hours on the floor with it playing with blocks and books and watching Disney cartoons. It will create bizarre, abstract drawings for you to stick on your fridge and say great stuff such as "Why aren't I a tree?" It will get dressed up as a giant cheese for school play night. You will tie its shoes and make thousands of sandwiches and carrot sticks for its lunch. On Father's Day, it will make you cold tea and burnt toast and present you with the most hideous and aesthetically unappealing hand-painted coffee mug in the history of mankind, and yet you will be strangely proud of it and treat it with the utmost respect and value. For years. You will carry this now infinitesimally small spot on your shoulders around a zoo and find yourself making crazy animal noises for illustrative purposes. You will feel hopeful as you launch it on its bike for the first time without training wheels, exhilarated as it pedals off manically into the distance, concerned as it suddenly veers off and disappears down an embankment, and sheepish as you explain to your wife why your child now has four stitches in its forehead. You will spend hours throwing balls and kicking balls and hitting balls together at the park. You will teach it to drive a car and struggle not to grab the steering wheel every time a corner is taken too widely, and you will lie awake at night because it borrowed your car and is two hours late in getting home. You will treasure the photo you have of you and this spot on top of a mountain on your camping holiday. This little thing will take you to the peaks of pleasure ("I love you, Dad") and to the depths of despair ("Dad, I just backed the car into the side of the house"). And then, one day, that microscopic cell will leave home and you'll wonder what you ever did before it came along.

Morning Sickness

At this stage, you are probably still unaware you are travelling down the road to dadhood. It's not like there's an app on your phone that buzzes you with a message:

> CODE RED FERTILIZATION ALERT: OvumApp has identified a sperm signal matching your DNA that has fertilized a nearby ovum. Currently at eight cell divisions and counting. Please verify with external testing.

At least . . . I don't think there is. *Is there?*

Similarly, the stork doesn't wake you up in the morning by tapping on your bedroom window and squawking, "YOUR WIFE'S PREGNANT! BRAAA! YOUR WIFE'S PREGNANT! BRAAA!"

But there *is* a telltale sign. An early warning system, if you like. Its medical name is the grandiosely titled nausea gravidarum, but most people just refer to it as morning sickness.

I still remember the day Meredith accompanied me to get a haircut. The salon was half-full of women getting perms and rinses and other things out of my experience and beyond my comprehension. Everything was going fine until she unexpectedly leapt up and bolted into the bathroom at the rear of the shop. For the next few minutes, we all sat there perplexed by the cacophony of gurgling and gagging, beautifully amplified by the tiled walls and floor.

At the time, I assumed this sudden and violent illness was due to my substandard attempt at a chicken laksa the previous evening. I don't think I'd even heard of morning sickness before (does coconut milk even *go* off?). But that sickness was the trumpet blast that heralded the end of one era of my life and the approach of a new one.

If only I could have seen the writing on the wall. It would have said, "Your wife's pregnant! Run away! Run away!" But back then I was ignorant about such things. You see, on the *outside*, my wife looked fine and normal, just like she did every day. A lifetime of television clichés had taught me that pregnant women staggered around, they groaned in and out of chairs, were prone to bouts of irrational hysteria, wore ridiculously frumpy maternity tents and developed inexplicable middle-of-the-night cravings for cucumber ice-cream or pickled onions on toast. But my wife was slim and attractive and athletic, and she was wearing jeans and a T-shirt; ergo, she was *not* pregnant.

But, on the *inside*, that sperm and ovum combination was hard at work on its human cocktail. And you can't have another person starting to grow within your own personal body space without certain side effects. The presence of the fertilized egg causes the mother's body to be flooded with estrogen and hormones, including the insidious-sounding Beta hCG. Meredith's blood and major body systems had gone into overdrive. One small side effect was that she felt nauseous.

This is morning sickness, an unpleasant physiological reaction experienced by most pregnant women usually throughout their first three months. Think carsickness, or airsickness, or roller-coaster-after-a-seafood-lunch-and-a-few-pints sickness.

Then multiply the quease factor by ten. It got its rather obvious and uncreative name because of its unwelcome appearance in the early hours of the day, but in reality it can happen all day. It should really be called "24/7 sickness," but that doesn't really roll off the tongue as well.

There is only one positive aspect to morning sickness. Research suggests that women who suffer from it have fewer miscarriages, and it may be a sign that a fertilized egg has implanted successfully. However, while this quirky statistic may be of great interest and comfort to you, it is likely to be of little comfort to your wife as she throws up into a potted plant outside your local supermarket.

Confirming the Obvious

Some women know that they are pregnant within a few weeks of conception. Their biological systems start ringing alarm bells and they soon put two and two together. But you also hear stories about women who go to their doctor with suspected irritable bowel syndrome or a gallstone problem only to find their gallstone has eyes, hands and a heartbeat and is already eight months old. Obviously, their biological alarm bells did not ring loudly enough. They put two and two together but ended up with three.

However, quite a few moms have assured me that most women *know* when they are pregnant. "It's just one of those instinctive things," they say. Being a guy, I can't validate or refute this comment, but I guess there must come a point in every woman's pregnancy when she begins to suspect that something is going on down in the engine room. It might be because of a missed period or food cravings. It might be because her breasts have become sore or because she is suddenly moody or tired or in frequent need of a toilet. It might be because of an unexpected propensity to vomit, even when you didn't cook the night before. It may well even be "just one of those instinctive things."

Once the woman reaches this point, however, things really start to heat up. She can go to either the phramacy or the doctor to have her suspicions confirmed with a pregnancy test.

Ah, the marvels of modern medical science! This test is really quite amazing and is certainly worth seeing. It measures the level of Beta hCG secreted into the mother's urine because of the suspected internal guest. There are a couple of different tests available from your pharmacy but they all basically involve introducing urine to some type of test strip. Some tests are even done "mid-stream," for those who like to live on the wild side. Home-pregnancy tests are about ninety-nine percent accurate and are best done first thing in the morning.

Pregnancy test kits used to resemble a credit card. (Heck, we even used to keep them in our wallets as a conversation starter!) Potential Mom would sprinkle four or five drops of urine on one corner of the card (something well outside my skill set), which then seeped across to the other corner, passing through a little viewing window en route. Five minutes later, Potential Mom watched as a little cross appeared in the window, confirming her suspicions. Meredith showed me one that said, in no uncertain terms, we were going to be parents.

Nowadays, pregnancy tests are quicker and leaner, resembling a thermometer. This is a good thing, because you won't ever have that awkward moment in a liquor store where you try buying a six-pack of pale ale by swiping your pissy pregnancy card. Oh yeah, that's a moment.

And Now, the News

There are two types of fathers.

There are the fathers who *have been trying* with their wives to become fathers. "We've been *trying* now for about twelve months," he will pipe up cheerily over an after-work drink, euphemistically referring to the fact that he has been having sex a lot. His wife and he have talked it over and they have both been *trying* for a long time to get it all happening. In the parental blogosphere, this is called TTC (*trying to conceive*).

Some guys have just always known they wanted to have children. It's just part of their identity and an integral narrative in how they see their lives playing out. For some – the fortunate – this may come to pass without too much effort or stress. But for others, despite their best efforts, pregnancy remains elusive, for any number of biological reasons, such as your sperm motility (capability of moving), or if your wife is heading towards her forties.

This can be a very long, complicated, emotionally rocky and frustrating process, perhaps involving thermometers, calendars, expensive cycles of *in vitro* fertilization (IVF) and visits to that special doctor who gives you a specimen jar and says, "Third cubicle on the right, if you please," and ten minutes later you have to hand the clear, plastic receptacle over to the intern behind the counter. Oh, the joy. (One of my friends even got into "Ovulation Tracking," a medical service that monitors ovulation and calculates the best times for intercourse, but really just brings to mind images of a surveillance satellite (from any Michael Bay movie) zooming in on a woman's uterus from a thousand kilometers up.)

Anyway, the bottom line is that this type of guy and his wife have been TTC, working hard at getting pregnant, at becoming parents, mother and father, mom and dad. He is expectant and is keenly waiting, planning and hoping for those magically whispered words, *"Darling, I'm pregnant."*

Then there is the *other* type of father. He is the one who has *not* been trying to become a father. (However, this doesn't necessarily mean that he hasn't been having sex a lot, nor that he doesn't necessarily want kids.) Perhaps in the heat of passion he and his wife brushed aside the security of contraception. Perhaps the contraception failed. Maybe they forgot that sex causes children or they just thought *damn the torpedoes* and wanted to see what would happen.

Anyway, the bottom line is that *this* type of guy and his wife enjoyed sex largely for relational purposes, as opposed to specifically "extending the family tree" purposes. He is *not* expectant and is *not* keenly waiting, planning and hoping for those magically whispered words.

Now, these guys have two things in common:

* in just a few months, they will both become fathers
* there will come a day soon where this important fact is revealed to them.

At this point, they may have fairly distinct and different responses to the actual news that fatherhood is nigh. Let's examine the different scenarios.

Father Type I – the one who has been *trying* – receives a cryptic text from his wife in his lunchbreak: "Dnt make 2 many plans 4 end of year. See u tonite."

He is uncertain and curious about this, but can't help but wonder, *Could it be . . . ?* At odd moments during the day, he is sure he can hear wafting violins somewhere in the background.

Later that day: "So what's the deal?"

"Darling, I saw Dr. Lloyd this morning."

[Crescendo of violins. Counter-melody subtly and harmoniously introduced by cellos and violas.]

"You mean . . . ?"

"Yes, my love. The tests were . . . positive."

[Massive crescendo. Whole symphony joins in.]

"You mean . . . ?"

"Yes, my honey blossom pancake . . . you're going to be . . . [and then the magical words as the whole room starts to spin uncontrollably in soft focus, accompanied by beautiful orchestral themes and bursts of color] A DAD."

He experiences a sensation of being lifted off the ground. He soars above the trees and spins around among the clouds. Clutching his wife to him, he feels deep inner warmth and fulfillment. It is a beautiful moment, full of symphonies and fireworks, confetti and rainbows.

Father Type II – the one who has *not been trying* – has something of a different experience. On his lunchbreak, he receives a cryptic text from his wife: "Dnt make 2 many plans 4 end of year. See u tonite."

He is uncertain and curious about this, but can't help but wonder, *Could it be* . . . a month in Bali? But at odd moments during the day, he is sure he can hear the theme from *Jaws* somewhere in the background.

Later that day: "So what's the deal?"

"Darling, I saw Dr. Lloyd this morning."

[Crescendo of *Jaws* theme. Aggressive, discordant counter-melody suddenly introduced à la staccato crotchets from *Psycho*.]

"You mean . . . ?"

"I had some tests. They were positive."

[Massive crescendo of untuned violins, timpani, gamelan and other nastily percussive instruments.]

"You mean . . . ?"

"I'm pregnant. You're going to be . . . [and then the room spins sickeningly to the deafening chorus of cannons, breaking glass and sirens] A DAD."

The room lurches like at the end of a bad bachelor party. His head swims and his knees buckle. He clutches his wife to him, for stability. In a feeble attempt at speech, he produces only pathetic squeaks and gurgles.

In this situation, it is important for the moment to be handled delicately. For example, there are certain things that should not be said, such as:

- How did you let that happen?
- Sorry, did you just say, "I'm eggplant"?
- I've got practice.
- We can't afford it.
- What's for dinner?
- That's fine, but don't expect me to get involved.

By the way, when your wife says she's pregnant, DON'T – whatever you do, DON'T – say, "Oh, you better sit down," as if she's some sort of invalid. They only do that on TV.

If you're a Father Type I, you probably feel pretty good. You've been trying to be a parent and you've just found out that soon you will be, so everything's sweet.

If you're a Father Type II, your first reaction could be anywhere on the scale from mild surprise and delight to confusion, shock and possibly fear. Don't feel too bad. I've been a Father Type II three times now and it hasn't done me any harm (if you don't count those bouts of involuntary twitching). Meredith had been on the pill for a while, and for various and personal reasons, which are frankly none of your business, we decided that she should come off the pill. Our basic idea was that nature would take its course and she would fall pregnant eventually on some distant fantasy day in the future and, whenever that happened, it would be just fine.

It happened the next day.

Call me naive, but I thought that pregnancy was actually a pretty difficult thing to achieve and that our "nature's course" method would take a while. What I didn't know then was that there's a ballpark twenty percent chance that a sexually active couple can get pregnant in a given month, rising to about an eighty percent chance in a given year. As it so happened, Meredith and I turned out to be as fertile as the Nile Delta and only need to drink from the same coffee cup for her to start feeling sick in the morning.

I clearly remember the moment when I found out my life was about to take off in a new and radically unexpected direction. It was March 8. Meredith was picking me up from work. She'd needed the car that day because she was going to the doctor. She hadn't been her usual self since that emergency at the hairdresser's. It was a bit of a concern, really.

She waltzed in, looking totally cool and normal, and said hi. We engaged briefly in some light chat and then headed out through the drizzle that had plagued the city for the past few months. My mind was filled with thoughts of what we were going to have for dinner. Pizza? No, a chicken dish . . . or those Mexican things. What are they called?

"Pete, what are you doing on October 24?" asked she.

"Nothing," I replied, eyeing her sideways. "Why, what have you got in mind?"

Of course! *Tacos*.

"Parenthood," said she, with a mischievous grin.

Or are they *nachos*?

Parenthood.

Nachos.

Parenthood.

No, not *nachos*. The soft-wrap ones . . . um . . . yes, *burritos*!

Parenthood.

The word bounced around my cerebral cortex for a few seconds, trying desperately to find something to grasp onto, but all it found were recipes for guacamole and salsa. Toasted sandwiches, perhaps?

"I beg your pardon?" is what I meant to say, but my mouth mumbled something more along the lines of "E bed du plarnd?"

And there was that word again.

"Parenthood," she said. "I'm pregnant. We're going to be parents."

There was a moment's silence. Somewhere nearby, a magpie squawked.

"You're going to be a dad."

She smiled. Cool. Collected.

I wobbled. Shocked. Flushed.

Time stood still. I recall a ball of tumbleweed rolling past but, given the geographical unlikelihood of that, suspect I inserted this memory in retrospect.

A father.

The words slowly sank in.

A *father*? You mean a guy who wears socks with sandals and makes "dad jokes" at inopportune moments and who can't come to after-work drinks because he's got to get home to take little Jessie to taekwondo and we're so proud because Jessie got a certificate this week for being a good friend and helper at school?

ME? A *FATHER*? You mean like the guy on the expressway during school holidays, perched behind the wheel of a minivan filled to bursting with mattresses and assorted domestic detritus and screaming kids, with bikes swinging wildly on the racks, and through the fingerprint-encrusted window you can see that slightly crazed look on his face?

A father? Me? *My* father is a father! *His* father was a father! I'm only . . . a . . . a son. Worse, I'm just a boy, a child, a man-child, if you will. I've only just left home. I can't even iron my shirts properly. Panic! Changing diapers? Me?

Mayday . . . Mayday . . . I'm going down!!!!!! What about sleep? What about our mortgage? What about that overseas trip we were planning?

And what about dinner?

At this moment, one of my students passed by. "Hello, sir. How are you doing?" he piped up.

If only you knew, pal, I thought. *If only you knew.*

BTW, we had leftovers for dinner.

How Do Ya Feel?

This was my introduction to the wonderful world of fatherhood. One minute, I was coasting along through life at a happy pace. I was in control and was closely following "the plan." Our young married lives were progressing nicely and the bank balance told us we were finding our feet. We were starting to plan a backpacking trip through Europe. The next minute, it was all spinning madly out of control on a bizarre and unexpected tangent. Our future was suddenly plunged into the abyss of new and unexplored terrain.

Some men are thrilled and "over the moon" to hear the news of their impending dadhood. Some feel numb and uncertain. I felt a whole lot of emotions at once.

The first one was *guilt*. I felt guilty that I wasn't ecstatic. I felt guilty that I didn't rush forward and grab my wife and say "I love you," or something memorable like that. It wasn't like in the movies at all. Why didn't I feel . . . *paternal*? Where was the symphony orchestra? To be blunt, it took me a little while to warm to the idea.

In a way, I also felt *excited*. I didn't really know what lay ahead of me, but the news brought that kind of expectant, nervy thrill you get when something really big is about to happen, like when you were a kid lining up for a ride at the county fair while listening to the screams of fear from those already inside. Or that rush you get when you step through Customs into the unexplored terrain of a foreign country, so rich with promise.

I was struck dumb by the significance of the moment and felt that some philosophical and momentous words were in order. In a kind of slow-motion haze, I put my hand on Meredith's stomach and mumbled something grandiose about how, just inches away, under the skin, a new life was forming.

"No," she said, moving my hand, "just inches away under the skin is my bladder. The baby is . . . *here*."

Another feeling I had was *fear*. I felt it in the pit of my stomach and tasted it in my mouth. I was scared of this great big thing called *fatherhood*, now rushing inevitably towards me like a freight train. I was scared of the unknown. I knew absolutely nothing about babies. And I do mean *absolutely nothing*.

I never even liked holding other people's babies. Come to think of it, I still don't. I've always liked things to be neat and ordered (#OCD), and suddenly I was facing something way beyond my control.

It wasn't that I was *opposed* to the idea of becoming a father. I never planned *not* to be a father, if you know what I mean. It just took me by surprise. I mean, I didn't even suspect that Meredith was pregnant. To my mind, there was no subtle lead-up, no hints at what was to come. So I felt shocked and awkward that this was not another of our carefully laid, middle-class-young-upwardly-mobile-couple plans. I could not even begin to comprehend what the words "you're going to be a dad" meant. I knew how to teach *Hamlet* and how to cook a reasonable Tom Kha Gai. But be a dad? You must be kidding! It all seemed so big and scary.

So *life-changing*.

Since then, in chatting and corresponding with guys all over the place, I have discovered that this is not such an uncommon experience. It's all right to feel shock and guilt and the burden of responsibility. It's all right to feel inadequate and scared. Fatherhood *is* a big and scary prospect. It's not something that can be digested and dealt with in a few minutes, or learned by glancing through cute parent anecdotes from the *Reader's Digest* in your doctor's waiting room.

I would even go so far as to say that it's *good* for you to feel a bit anxious and a bit out of your depth. This at least shows that you are trying to process the whole thing and is a good motivator to action. I get more concerned when I meet guys who seem a bit cocky and casual, or shrug off impending fatherhood as something they'll just take in their stride without much thought or effort, like an apprentice carpenter who thinks he's a bit of a natural . . . until he loses a finger on a bandsaw.

The funny thing is, I spent a great deal of time considering what impact this new fatherhood thing was going to have on *my* life. But I'm embarrassed to say I didn't really consider at the time what Meredith might have been thinking about it all. Don't be so self-indulgent that you forget your wife is actually *having* the baby. She may well be feeling the same way. On top of which, she has the added anxiety of disruption to her work and nine months of increasing bodily discomfort, only to be topped off by the turmoil of birth, midnight breastfeeds and months of sheer exhaustion afterwards.

So talk with your wife. Discuss your fears, feelings and concerns. Share your expectations and ideas. Communicating and sorting out your feelings is a great way to establish the team philosophy of parenting, even at this early stage.

And remember, there's comfort in numbers. Bear in mind the fact that nearly every dad you know (including your own dad) probably felt just as out of their depth as you do. Not one single dad alive was born into the role; it is a role you grow into. Bit by bit. Day by day. And if the millions of other guys on the planet can do it, then odds are on that you can too, unless there's something *really* wrong with you.

Nobody expects you to be an instantaneous parenting expert. Even if you are totally ignorant and hopeless with kids, it doesn't matter. You'll learn.

I sure did.

You'll be surprised at how little time it takes to get used to the idea of fatherhood. And once you've recovered from the shock, it's time to start taking action.

There's much to be done and only a few months to go.

Let's Go Public

So where does that leave you now? To summarise, you have:

- had child-producing sex
- found out that your baby will enter the world in a few months
- recovered from the initial shock.

The next stage can be pleasant or traumatic, depending on:

- how you handle it
- whether or not your wife's family and friends actually *like* you.

I'm talking about *breaking the news* to people.

Encountering the various reactions of family and friends – screams, fainting, hysterical laughter, weeping, muscle failure, nonchalance, concern, and so on – can be a source of great amusement and the topic of dinnertime storytelling for years to come. But before you go telling everyone your news, there are a few things you should keep in mind.

First, don't go public too early in the piece. Miscarriage is not uncommon, especially in the first twelve weeks of a pregnancy, and that's something you probably only want your most inner circle of friends and family to know about. In addition, it is important that you and your wife have a bit of space to get used to the idea of becoming parents. There's no rush. Once the cat's out of the bag, people will look at you differently. Friends will want to give you advice and talk about parenting ad nauseam and have you over for dinner and start knitting little jackets and booties. Your conversations will be dominated by annoying questions and lengthy anecdotes ranging from the horrific ("Did we tell you about Sal's emergency Caesarean?") through the disgusting ("Anyway, Scottie pulled his diaper off in the car and when we stopped two hours later the entire back seat was smeared with . . .") to the plain mind-numbing ("But listen, one of the best features of this stroller is this little Velcro tab here. See this Velcro tab? Watch what happens when I pull it . . ."). Your friends and relatives will cease to look at you as "a couple"; you will become "parents-to-be."

So you and your wife should stew over it for a while to get a bit more comfortable with the whole idea. Treasure your moments together as "a couple."

Second, news about impending parenthood spreads faster than a virus in a zombie-apocalypse movie. Thanks to the light speed of the internet and ubiquitous social media, from the time you break the news to the first person, it only takes forty-five seconds for every single person you've ever met in your entire life to find out that you're going to be a dad. You pull into a service station and the guy at the pump next to you – who you swear you've never met before – winks at you and says, "Hey, man, I heard your wife's eating for two. Congratulations!" If you want to tell people yourself instead of letting them hear it on the e-grapevine, you have to time the announcement with the speed and precision of a military operation. If you don't, the surprise will be spoiled and everyone will know.

Third, there are familial and peer politics to consider. In some families, there is a "pecking order," and if you don't pay heed to it you may end up paying the price for the rest of your life. You know what I'm talking about. If you tell your neighbor before you tell your mother-in-law, there will be hell to pay. Like an elephant, she will never forget. (Just let me make it clear at this point that in no way do I consider *my* mother-in-law to be in any way like an elephant.)

Anyway, one of the best things about good news is telling other people. There are some people you will want to tell face to face (immediate family and friends within geographical reach); others you will want to tell in person (phone calls or Skype with distant family and friends); and only then should you unleash your news into the viral wilderness of social media.

First, our parents. We sat them down on the couch. With the benefit of hindsight, I could have handled it better. Not knowing how to broach the subject subtly, I jabbed a finger at Meredith and, with a look on my face like a naughty school-boy, blurted out, "She's pregnant!"

My mother did a little involuntary dance, then she went off to put the kettle on. My dad, repeating his performance from the day we announced our engagement, sat there flapping his jaw and wearing a glazed expression on his face. When he stirred himself into action, moments later, he pulled Meredith onto his knee and mumbled, "You better sit down."

My mother-in-law was pretty cool about the whole thing. We told her in the hallway of her apartment as she came home from work laden with groceries. She didn't even drop anything.

Then we told my ninety-year-old great-aunt. "WE ARE HAVING A BABY!" I yelled into her hearing aid.

"No, no gravy for me, thank you," she said.

Next, our friends. One leapt screaming across a table at us while her husband had a small seizure. Another group of friends immediately broke out the warm bubbly. One friend suddenly developed lockjaw, and all he could do was repeat guttural sounds.

While social media allows you to simply tweet or post your news to all and sundry, I like the subtlety of a zany photo, with my "Top Three" being, for no immediately discernible reason:

1. Photograph of couple holding a sign with arrow pointing to woman's abdomen, stating "Coming Soon" (and then the date). A variation on this is the abdomen close-up with one of those rear-window car signs stuck on it: "BABY ON BOARD."
2. Photograph of what are obviously men's shoes (clichéd dirty boots), women's shoes (clichéd stilettoes) and baby booties, all in a row.
3. Photograph of the "positive" home-pregnancy-testing stick.

Post it without comment, and watch the fun and games unfold.

When using social media to declare your good news, remember this one important truth. Babies are good news. Pregnancy makes people happy. Your friends will be thrilled to hear you are having a baby. However, after posting your news, please do not misconstrue your 187 "likes" as an invitation from your "friends" to now engage in a daily tsunami of pregnancy and baby updates, tweets, posts and photos. Failure to heed this advice will see your friends clicking "unfollow" faster than you can type "multi-nucleated syncytiotrophoblast."

Myth Busting

Before we go any further with our exploration of fatherhood, now is as good a time as any to bust some myths. Many of the expectations that I had as a new father turned out to be pure fiction. As a consequence, paternal reality turned out to be something of a slap in the face. Why? Because a main source of information about many facets of the universe is what we see in movies.

Unfortunately, movies are an unreliable teacher across a whole range of human endeavor. A lot of what you see in movies regarding *life* only takes place in the magical fantasy of a scriptwriter's head. If you believe that what you see on the screen is reality, you will end up in trouble.

For example, regarding sex. When I got married, I had an adolescent expectation that when I got home after a hard day's work, my negligee-clad wife would greet me at the door with a glass of champagne in her hand and a rose clamped between her teeth. Each night would herald a candlelit feast, followed by nocturnal pleasures on an epic scale.

The movies lied.

The same applies to violence. In your average mega-budget action flick, the protagonist will get shot at with thousands of bullets, rockets, bombs and lasers, pushed off cliffs, punched through walls, fall down elevator shafts, survive their car somersaulting through buildings, jump from planes and choppers and get pounded by the fists, feet and weapons of multiple muscled thugs or martial arts bad guys or evil aliens, yet end up with just a dishevelled hairdo, a slight smirk and some torn sexy clothing. In the real world, however, when I reach for my shopping bags at an awkward angle, I put my back out and I'm off work for three days.

Again, the movies lied.

Movies also paint a different picture than reality about pregnancy, birth and fatherhood. Real-life pregnant women don't always stagger around groaning with their hands on their hips, and they don't need to sink awkwardly into a chair after every few steps. While food cravings are a normal part of pregnancy, they generally do not result in a 2 am emergency run to your local 24-hour grocery for licorice and sauerkraut. It is unlikely that your drive to the hospital when your wife is in labor will be a high-speed, red-light-busting comedy of errors with a police escort. Odds are on that your wife won't be pushed down the hospital corridor on a wheelie bed while you run alongside clutching her hand and declaring your undying love. Women rarely give birth with their feet up in stirrups, and I'm sorry to disappoint you but you probably won't get to wear a gown, booties and surgical mask for the labor. Also absent will be the witty repartee between you and your wife as she grunts comically to push the baby out. And gone now is the hospital practice of lining up the recent newborns behind a plate-glass window for all the relatives to stare at like pasteries displayed in a cake shop. And, if you try lighting a celebratory cigar in a hospital waiting room, you'll be beaten by nurses with bedpans.

If you're looking to TV shows or movies to supply you with a paternal role model, don't bother (See Appendix I: Parental Education Films). TV and movie dads tend to fall into one of two categories, both of which are equally ineffectual and pathetic.

On the one hand, there is the Superdad. He has an understanding smile and incredible wisdom. He solves all problems with a few paternal clichés and the family is better again. He is always in control and is always selfless and giving, and work never seems to impinge on the plentiful time he has to devote to family. Of course, you never see these dads make a bed, change a diaper, set the table or lose their temper.

On the other hand, there is the *anti-dad*. These dads are ridiculously inept at fathering. They have no domestic or relational skills, and are often selfish and morally questionable. They have terrible relationships with their kids and treat them either as cuddly toys or with a sense of vague or comedic detachment.

But movies aren't entirely to blame for this constant stream of lies. The same applies to many parenting books, particularly the big ones with lots of glossy photos. I'm not sure where exactly these photos are taken, but it's not Earth. Maybe it's that fantasy world known as Bookland, a place of perpetual political correctness and saccharine soft focus.

In Bookland, pregnant women float about in flattering pastel outfits. They spend their days with their hands resting meaningfully on their abdomens and wearing soft, warm, contemplative expressions on their faces. Their Bookland square-jawed husbands (who look like buff and tanned models from advertisements for precision watches or aftershave) hold their wives tenderly and stare deeply into their eyes. Bookland dads are especially good at assembling cribs and car seats without losing their tempers or slipping a disc.

In Bookland, laboring women don't sweat. They merely look determined. Their serious but competent and well-dressed husbands support them by knowing exactly what they want and giving it to them. The women give birth to remarkably clean three-month-old babies on crisp sheets *sans* blood and other fluids. Sometimes, the babies don't even have umbilical cords. All is laughter and tears of joy and sincerity.

Of course, the stars of the Bookland fantasy are the Superbabies – babies that perpetually smile, gurgle and cock their heads like cute puppies. Their eyes are alert, their skin is perfect and their heads are the way heads should be. Incredibly, their diapers are totally devoid of unsightly substances.

It's also worth being slightly wary of women's magazines, which for many pregnant women are one of the five basic food groups. These have a tendency to normalize the "my miracle baby" stories . . . you know, where women over fifty have an amazing IVF birth experience (despite their eighty percent chance of miscarriage) or where the baby born at twenty-three weeks still survived. They provide an artificial and unrealistic hope that my baby too might be that "one in a million" baby, fuelled by the experiences of some pop diva or B-grade soap star.

Don't even get me started on the internet.

So, as you walk the parental road, don't spend too much time comparing your own mixed-up world with the perfection so often served up in books, movies, magazines, or on TV or the net.

That will only make you feel bad.

Congratulations

So, you're going to be a dad.

Congratulations. Have a cigar. Take the day off work. Have a few friends raise a glass in your honor. But, while not wanting to spoil the moment here, exactly *why* should *you* be congratulated? No offense, but what exactly have you done to date that is worthy of all this back-patting, huh?

In short, you had sex. That's all you've done. Chipped in a lucky sperm, enjoyable as it was. It's something that millions of humans and animals do every day, including that gang of annoying cats outside my bedroom window.

Essentially, you can become a dad as a side effect of a brief moment of sexual pleasure. This concept is declared in Ron Howard's quirky film *Parenthood*, when a young Keanu

Reeves says to Dianne Wiest in a brash surfer-dude accent, "You know . . . you need a license to buy a dog or drive a car. Hell, you need a license to catch a fish. But they'll let any asshole be a father."

To become a teacher, it took me four years of university study. To drive a car, I took lessons and had to pass theoretical and practical tests. To be a father, however, all I needed was an erection, my wife and a few glasses of wine.

This logic seems backward to me, considering that becoming a dad is infinitely more important and significant than learning about visual literacy or knowing how far away from a stop sign you can park your car. Any man with a working appendage can become a *biological parent*. But becoming a *good dad* takes considerably more time and effort. Donating the sperm was the easy part. All the hard work – and all the good stuff – lies ahead of you.

You don't suddenly and mystically start wearing the "Dad cap" on the day your child is born. Don't wait that long to start working on becoming a father. If you keep waiting for the "right time," it will never come. Consider the next few months as the training ground where you get to warm up and prepare for fatherhood.

You don't want to end up like the dad in the classic Harry Chapin song "Cat's in the Cradle," who was always too busy to spend time with his son. One day, he woke up and realized that his son had grown up, but by then it was too late. This is a great song, one that has on occasion reminded me what my life is about. I must admit, though, I have never quite fathomed exactly what the cat was doing in the cradle in the first place, to say nothing of the song's blatant disregard of the inherent dangers of toxoplasmosis.

Anyway, I'm sidetracking. Back to the heavy stuff.

Being a dad – being a *good* dad – is really important. It is a huge responsibility and a wonderful joy and a mammoth commitment. But here's the thing. It doesn't start when your child is old enough to catch a ball in the backyard. It doesn't start when it utters its first words or takes its first steps. It doesn't even start the first time you hold it.

It starts *now*.

It starts while your baby is still a mere cluster of cells in the womb. It's vital that you get your head together early in the piece and establish good patterns in fathering. So, if you want to be a good dad – an involved dad – start *now*.

Congratulations on having been given the privilege and responsibility of becoming a father. But if you want to smoke the cigar, earn the right.

2

Pregnancy

"They've got to get themselves from being a single cell
to a whole person complete with a full set of functioning
body parts, without instructions or an allen key.
Now that's an achievement."

Sugar and Spice . . .

Some people have a gift for asking the stupid question.

Such as, on your birthday: "Do you feel any older?"

Or on the return from your honeymoon: "How's married
life treating you?"

Or when your wife says: "What do you think of my new
skirt?"

Or when your aunt hasn't seen you in a while: "My, you're
tall, aren't you?"

Stupid.

Being in the baby-making game does not exclude you
from such wanton conversational stupidity. The question I was

constantly asked during each of Meredith's pregnancies was "What do you think you're having: a boy or a girl?"

This is a stupid question. On two fronts.

First, your child's sex is a lucky dip. You get what you get and there is simply no way of intuitively perceiving whether it's going to be a boy or a girl. Sure, there may be a genetic disposition in your family, like friends of mine whose family line produced only boys for ninety-nine years. And some couples take either natural or technical steps to try to manipulate the sex of their child, such as eating fresh pineapple before conceiving under a full moon while facing south and reciting the *Bhagavad Gita*. But, for most couples, the sex of their child is as good as the flip of a coin.

Second, it doesn't matter what you *think* anyway. You can *think* whatever you like and even *hope* whatever you like but ultimately this has no bearing on whether you're having a boy or a girl. You can *think* your wife is going to give birth to a wheel of camembert and it still won't make an iota of difference.

However, this segues nicely into the more interesting question of whether or not you should, or even *can*, find out the sex of your unborn child. One really reliable method is to dangle your gold wedding ring on a string over your wife's belly and if the ring swings in a clockwise rotation then . . . hang on, did I say "reliable"? My apologies. I meant to say "crazy old wives' tale." Silly me.

It is common for women to have a few scans during their pregnancy, some of which might provide an indication of your child's gender. There is one early on to try to vagin-angulate your baby's due date. (Don't bother looking up that word. I just made it up.) Then, around three months in, there's the impressive-sounding nuchal scan (which gets its name *not*, as you might have expected, from the incredibly impressive Doctor Nuchal in the 1800s, but because the scan looks at the nape of the baby's neck to identify possible congenital issues with the developing fetus). And then, around twenty weeks in, there is the fetal anomaly scan, which seeks to make sure all the bits of your baby are doing what you hope they would do (i.e. ten fingers, two kidneys, one head, no gills, etc.).

By the time your wife has the second of these ultrasounds, a few months in, the trained eye of the radiographer will be able to pick out subtleties in the scan (i.e. the presence or absence of a penis, or, more precisely, the delightfully titled "genital nub") that will indicate to them – with pretty good but not flawless accuracy – the sex of your child. They will usually ask if you want to know.

We decided *not* to find out. We liked the excitement and suspense of not knowing. We were happy to wait till the big day itself when the midwife would present our newborn to us and say, "Congratulations, Dr. and Mrs. Downey, what have you got there?" It felt somehow, that *not* knowing was more traditional, the way births have been for centuries, and in some whimsical way that appealed to us. (Besides, *not* knowing gives dad a job to do at the birth.)

I have only a few friends who confirmed the sex of their child beforehand. One wanted to know because she wanted to deck out the nursery and start buying clothes in appropriate colors. ("Gender stereotyping!" I growled at her and made a mental note to buy her unborn daughter a toy bulldozer for her first birthday.) Another wanted to know because she already had four sons and desperately wanted a daughter and couldn't bear the suspense. If she was going to be "disappointed," she wanted to deal with the "disappointment" earlier rather than later (although how anyone could be "disappointed" with a healthy baby – boy or girl – is beyond me). Another wanted to know so they could pick a name. And another friend found out – even though she didn't want to – when the radiographer slipped up while looking at a scan and said, "Oh look, he's sucking his thumb!"

Anyway, have a chat about this with your wife and work out what you want to do.

And while I'm on the topic of stupid parenting questions, people still ask me if, as the father of three daughters, I am desperate for a son. Well, the answer is no, I'm not. I like having girls. At least they don't shoot jets of urine into your face while you're changing their diapers. Besides, everyone knows that girls are made of sugar and spice and all things nice, whereas boys are made of frogs and snails and puppy-dog tails, which is disgusting.

I just hope that, if my daughters get married, our society will have lost its antiquated assumption that the father of the bride has to pay for the wedding. Because if it hasn't, the only wedding presents my daughters will get from me will be a ladder and a suitcase each.

Having said that, I wouldn't have minded having a boy, either. We could have done macho stuff together, like chopping down trees and painting murals on the side of his panel van. And I would have looked forward to the day of his marriage because it sure wouldn't have been me who'd be paying for it. Everyone knows that's the father of the bride's responsibility.

Internal Growth

Much of the kerfuffle surrounding this whole *childbirth thang* is directed at the moms, and, to a lesser extent, us dads. The pages of many books, magazines and websites are directed at all the emotional, social, physical and psychological changes that we parents need to make in taking on our destined roles in life. This is to say nothing of all the parental – and, if you're really unlucky, *grand*-parental – advice that will be coming your way.

You will be busy trying to adjust mentally to fatherhood, you will be racing to baby-proof your home, and you will be exhausted from shopping for all the necessities. But in the midst of all this busy-ness and self-indulgence, we can sometimes begin to forget the star of the show: the baby.

If you think *you've* got problems trying to get your stuff together in only nine months, imagine how the baby feels. They've got to get themselves from being a single cell to a whole person complete with a full set of functioning body parts, without instructions or an allen key. Now *that's* an achievement.

So let's put things back in perspective. The last time we mentioned the baby, the sperm had just connected with the ovum up there in the Fallopian tube and it had started its nine-month journey towards birth into the outside world.

But what happens in the interim?

Up to the point when Meredith first said to me those memorable words "You're going to be a dad," I really knew very little about what actually went on in the uterus, or "womb." (By the way, I have always disliked that word. It sounds too goofy for such an important part of the body and brings to mind the noise made by a returning boomerang – *womb womb womb womb womb*.) As a teenager studying biology at high school, I was a lot more interested in soccer stars, skateboards and guitar chords than the technicalities of fertility.

With the birth of our first child imminent, I consulted a few textbooks from my university days, but the technical words were enough to drive me back into ignorance. The same applied for the cross-section diagrams of female reproductive passages shown at birth class.

But then, just before Rachael was born, I came across some awe-inspiring and groundbreaking (albeit controversial) photos by acclaimed photographer Lennart Nilsson revealing the previously hidden world of the womb. Suddenly, a light bulb flashed somewhere above my head. The veil of ignorance was lifted and the miracle of life became clear at last.

So, for all of you unversed in the biological intricacies of pregnancy, here is the layman's version:

Mr. Tadpole swims down the tunnel and . . . um . . .

Once the sperm and ovum have combined, the sex of your child has been determined, depending on whether the sperm is an X sperm (girl) or a Y sperm (boy). The chromosomes and genes within the sperm and ovum have also set all of the child's genetic information: the length of its fingers, the shape of its eyes, the arrangement of its teeth, the color of its nasal hair and even the diseases it will inherit. These have all been decided and blueprinted into the growth sequence of the cells. This genetic program can be dominated by the features and traits of you or your wife or any of your ancestors. This does not, however, explain why most babies look like Winston Churchill when they are born.

Within a day of fertilization, the nucleus will split, and continue to split again and again in an exponential growth process. About five days after fertilization, the thing that will in a few months be your child is still officially – and again rather unromantically – called a blastocyst. This is a very important developmental stage because it is here that the cells start forming into different structures; the outside of the blastocyst is a hollow sphere of cells (the cool-sounding trophoblast), which will in time form the cocoon-like placenta, where your child will grow for the next several months. Clinging inside that is a cluster of cells (the also cool-sounding embryoblast) which will in time grow into an embryo, which is, in short, your child.

Again, you just have to stop sometimes and think *wow*.

The blasto will begin to move south down the Fallopian tube on a three-day journey to the uterus, where it will bob around for a while looking for a cozy spot to "dig in." It is choosy about this, and may take up to three days before it comes across a satisfactory spot to set up camp. Once it implants, conception has officially occurred and the Beta hCG hormone will be produced, signalling to the mother that she is pregnant, through the gift of morning sickness.

The now embryo will then continue to split and grow until, at about the one-week mark, it will closely resemble a tiny sea anemone. It will sprout and mutate in many different directions before it even vaguely begins to look human. Two weeks from conception, it will look like something from a seafood platter, and at about the one-month mark, like that hideous beast from *Alien*, it will have a seahorse-like tail and elongated head.

All the time, this fleshy blob will develop a brain, nerves, bones, blood vessels, muscles, intestines, a heart and massive vocal cords (for late-night screaming). Six weeks after fertilization, arms and legs will appear and a tiny heart will start beating at 150 beats a minute. Fingers grow. The lens, cornea and iris of the eye take shape. And all of this happens automatically, without any intervention or strategic planning on your part, something that in the middle of a sleepless night will have you contemplating the wonder of life and your infinitesimally small place in an infinitely complex universe.

By the end of the third month, the embryo will have graduated to the dizzy heights of being a *fetus*. You could hold this fetus in the palm of your hand. It even looks human, sort of – although I certainly wouldn't want to bump into one on a dark night.

And that's your child. Minuscule, yes. A little weird-looking, yes. But give it time. It still has six months to go.

During these months, the fetus will float in warm, salty fluid in a cocoon called the amniotic sac, inside the mother's uterus. Growing and living in an enclosed, aquatic environment raises certain puzzling questions. Namely:

- How does the fetus breathe?
- How does the fetus get food?
- How does the fetus get rid of its waste?

In actual fact, the fetus (or baby, if you like) does not use its mouth at all for oxygen or food consumption, and it doesn't use its bum for waste expulsion. This is a good thing, for obvious reasons. The secret lies in technology developed by the Russians in 1965 for the Voskhod 2 spacewalk. Astronauts walking in space use a hollow, hose-like tether called an *umbilical cord* to receive all their necessary life-support requirements from the mothership. Women have taken this technology on board and now utilize it in their wombs (*womb womb womb womb . . .*).

The mother breathes air and eats food, and all the good stuff necessary for life is absorbed into her bloodstream. The nutrients are transferred to the baby through a halfway station where the amniotic sac and the uterine wall meet. This is called the placenta. Although the baby in its sac has its own blood supply and there is negligible exchange of blood itself, all the life-support materials (oxygen, vitamins, carbohydrates, minerals, etc.) soak through the placenta and travel down the umbilical cord straight into the baby's blood supply. Other things that can travel down the umbilical cord are nicotine, alcohol, garlic and wi-fi. The baby's wastes leave through a separate channel down the same cord.

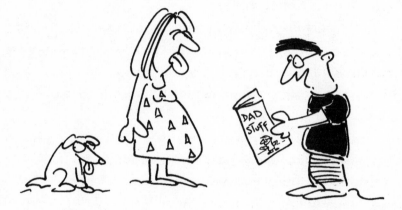

One interesting and exciting feature of all this growth is that, as the baby gets bigger, it starts doing stuff. It sucks its thumb. It dreams (although one wonders what it dreams about, given its limited life experiences). It moves around, turns, kicks, punches, stretches. Basically, it's looking for a way out of there.

For most dads, getting to feel their child kick is a real thrill that makes them realize for the first time that there really is a little person in there. Most babies, however, have a sixth sense, so that even if they are constantly busting out some Muay Thai moves, as soon as their father puts his hand out to feel them, they freeze.

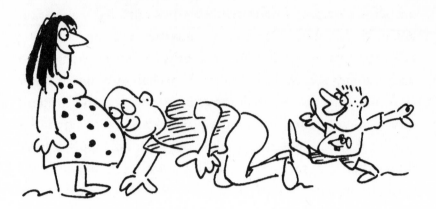

Here's to Her Health!

Since the baby is developing and growing inside the mother, it stands to reason that the health and general wellbeing of the mother will have a direct effect on the health and wellbeing of the baby. In short, it is important that the mother stays healthy during the pregnancy.

In no way do I wish to imply that you are in charge of your wife's health. She is a free spirit, an adult who makes her own decisions. But while she is responsible for her health, it's good to know things that you can do to help.

In terms of diet, a good range of fresh food is essential to provide both mother and baby with all the necessary bits from the pyramid of food groups. Healthy and tasty home-cooked and prepared meals are going to trump doughnuts, fizzy drinks, chips and a Triple Deluxe Ultimate Extreme Burger every time, so take it easy on the junk.

Drugs have a direct impact on the unborn. If you ever go to the pharmacy for supplies, always inform the pharmacist that your medications are for a pregnant woman, and read the manufacturer's directions on the side of the box. You will be surprised at how many everyday drugs, from worm tablets to antihistamines, are "not suitable for pregnant women." Then again, in this era of litigo-caution, pretty much everything is labelled as being unsuitable for pregnant women – including stuff they give you in hospitals – in the same way that every cookie nowadays seems to "contain traces of nuts." Just in case. (And, speaking of worms and germs and things, your wife should avoid eating rare or raw meat and handling cat or dog feces because of a disease called toxoplasmosis. It will no doubt be a great disappointment to her to discover that she will have to stay away from pet excrement for several months, but, hey, we all have to make sacrifices.)

One of the challenges for a pregnant woman can be not drinking alcohol. It wasn't that long ago that light and occasional drinking was considered okay, maybe even healthy, for the pregnant woman. And, of course, there was always the anecdotal evidence of somebody's aunt who drank like a fish while she was pregnant, and her kids turned out okay (with the exception of cousin Derek). But those days are over.

Pretty much every baby and health organization with a fancy title and logo will err on the side of caution and say that not enough is known about pregnancy and alcohol, and therefore alcohol should be avoided altogether. Pregnant women who drink run the risk of giving birth to a child with a fetal alcohol spectrum disorder (FASD). The more they drink and the more frequently, the greater the risk. This makes sense, given that, essentially, when a pregnant woman drinks, her baby drinks too, due to the transference through the placenta. So if you and your wife are in the habit of having a drink together or are connoisseurs of fine wines, perhaps you can help by not cracking a bottle of Domaine de la Romanée – Conti La Tâche over dinner.

The same applies to smoking. Smoking is *really* bad news for an unborn because the baby can't get all the oxygen it needs at the critical time when it really needs it. Of course, I don't need to tell you this. Everyone knows smoking is bad, but if you're addicted, giving up is not as simple as reading a few comical or guilt-tripping words in a book like this. (Smokers: please allow me a non-pious plea to do whatever you can and elicit whatever support you need to give up smoking during pregnancy and the baby years. You can do it, and it will really make a difference for your baby. A really big difference. And now, I will go back to being pious . . .)

Cigarettes are packed full of junk that your baby most definitely does not want to know about, including ammonia, nicotine, tar, formaldehyde, nickel, cadmium, carbon monoxide and even poisons (arsenic and cyanide) and radioactive compounds. This can lead to a whole panoply of problems, the least of which is stunted fetal development, which in turn leads to reduced birth weight. Smoking also increases the potential for miscarriage, deformity and, in severe cases, the death of the baby soon after birth. The child of a smoking mother is twice as likely to die of sudden infant death syndrome (SIDS), and this risk doubles again if the father smokes. Cigarette packs are not kidding when they state "Smoking harms your unborn baby."

If you and your wife smoke and she decides to give it up, respect and support her by not smoking near her, because *passive smoking* is also dangerous (#Duh). Don't smoke while she's trapped in the car or in an unventilated room with you. Smoke chemicals are also transferred through skin and clothing, so maybe have a "smoking jacket" that you can put on and take off before handling your baby. A smoking jacket is, traditionally, a mid-thigh-length velvet or silk robe (although both materials can be sported at once) with a fancy lining and festooned with large toggles or buttons. Which is pretty lucky for you, 'cause I'm sure you've got one or two of those bad boys lying around. But if you don't, a hoodie or track jacket top will be fine. Apart from that, wash your hands before you touch your baby.

Then again, maybe you could even give it up yourself? If you can't give it up, perhaps you could move to Norway.

Decisions, Decisions

The thing about pregnancy is that the baby won't stay in there forever. It has to come out sometime. When it does come out, the process is called labor, which brings up images of hard or fatiguing work, kind of like spending a day digging in the garden or laying concrete. This is a great euphemism; a word such as *agony* is probably more appropriate to describe the process of childbirth, but let's face it: who would want to end up in an *Agony Ward*?

Women have been giving birth for millions of years. Um . . . well, technically speaking, millions of years ago they probably weren't "women" in the way you and I might conceive of them. Let's just say . . . "females." Whatever. The main point is that childbirth has been going on since Year Zero. It is a natural and normal part of our life cycle. My guesstimate is that 99.9 percent of these births throughout history took place in fairly mundane circumstances – in the field, the cave, the shelter, the back room, the hut, the weatherboard house, the isolated farmhouse – possibly attended by a local "expert," generally an older woman or women experienced in and not freaked out by the holy ritual of childbirth. Fortunately, in our modern world, there are a lot more specialist facilities and professional personnel at your disposal to help you and your wife navigate the pregnancy and the birth safely.

And so, fairly early in the pregnancy, you and your wife will need to make some decisions about:

- what professional/s you are going to employ to assist you through the whole shebang
- how and where the labor and birthing process is going to take place.

This is because, like many other good things in life – overseas trips and a night at the theater, for example – you just can't sort it out on the day. You need to plan ahead.

Midwife or Obstetrician?

Midwives have been around since year zero. Even four thousand years ago, historical evidence points to the existence of the professional birth attendant – the midwife – who had training and skill in assisting women to navigate the birth process. In fact, the term midwife actually comes from Old English *midwyf*, meaning "with-woman." The modern midwife is a highly specialized and trained healthcare practitioner who supervises and cares for women during pregnancy, labor, birth and after the birth. They work in home, birth-center and hospital contexts.

An obstetrician is a medical doctor, a surgeon who has specialized in the field of obstetrics/gynecology. They are experts in the female reproductive system who monitor their patients during pregnancy and are able to make medical or surgical interventions in the case of birth complications. Obstetricians have a lot of letters after their name and drive convertibles with speedometers that go up to 260 miles an hour.

Obstetricians and midwives often work in tandem. They don't work across every hospital, but rather are connected with particular hospitals, so that may be another factor limiting your wife's choice. And, like a hospital, their time is finite, so she'll have to schedule with them as well. Once again, this needs to be done fairly quickly. Like, tomorrow. In relation to midwives and obstetricians, there are a few options.

Option 1: Your Own Obstetrician

You essentially choose and employ your own obstetrician, paying a fee for appointments and for the birth and postnatal care. There are insurance discounts available, but it can still be costly. The woman can give birth in birth centers or hospitals where the obstetrician has "visiting rights," which can include private and public hospitals. She is cared for in labor by nurses, and her obstetrician will come in for the birth and a quick postnatal check-up for the first few days. (Except in the case of our Georgia, who was in a hurry to get into the world, so the obstetrician didn't make it in time and it was all done by the hospital midwives.) Obstetricians may be advisable if there are potential birth complications, such as in the case of some older mothers or women with medical conditions or physical issues.

Option 2: Your Own Midwife

Like the obstetrician, you essentially choose and employ your own midwife, paying a fee for appointments and for the birth and postnatal care. Health plans offer some assistance with midwife fees; just make sure the midwife is in your network. The woman can give birth at home or at a stand-alone birth center. If complications arise, the midwife can either take the woman to a hospital where she has visiting rights and therefore continue care, or to any hospital, where she hands over official care to a hospital-based midwife but continues providing care as a "professional support person." These private midwives may not have professional indemnity insurance, which makes this option more complex and expensive but generally is your best choice for a home birth.

Option 3: Hospital-Based Midwifery
This is where midwifery care is provided not privately but through a hospital. The woman contacts the hospital or birth center in her area (there are usually only one to three to choose from, depending on the area) and requests an appointment with a midwife, or she may need to call an outpatient center. Ask or check the hospital's website. The woman will have care from one or perhaps two midwives for her prenatal appointments, and a midwife will be on call for her birth, to provide care to her in labor and during birth. Doctors in the hospital are on standby but are not involved in the care unless medical complications arise. This is certainly a good option in terms of the advantages that come with continuity of care. (This would be our preferred option if we were to have our time again or have more kids. Even though we are *not* having any more kids, thank you very much.)

Midwives will see the woman in the hospital during the short stay following the birth and also in a health center setting in the weeks and months after birth. The midwife will check on the woman's health, provide assistance with breastfeeding, and emotional support, and talk about contraception and family planning options. The mother-to-be has a lot of flexibility with appointments and care with midwives, but as there may be a variety of midwives caring for her at the hospital, she won't get the same continuity as with one obstetrician.

Option 4: GP-Shared Care
The woman has her antenatal appointments with her local doctor (GP), has three appointments at the hospital to make sure everything is ready for birthing at the hospital and is cared for by a nurse who is on for that shift in the delivery ward, and then by nurses postnatally. The woman has continuity antenatally but may not receive much labor or birth education, and will not have met the nurse caring for her in labor or postnatally (which is often the same case for Option 3). This is a popular option for baby number two as the mothers feel they don't need as much pregnancy education.

Selecting a Midwife or Obstetrician
If you choose to employ your own obstetrician or midwife, how do you go about selecting them?

It may be that your wife already has one. But, if she doesn't, she has to shop for one. I have a friend who visited four obstetricians and then chose the one she liked best. Shopping around like this offers maximum choice, but it also promises to be expensive. Don't do it unless at least one of you is an international business tycoon.

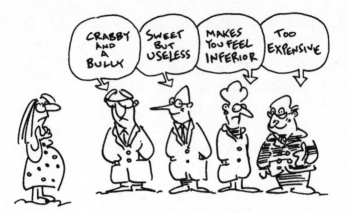

Most of my friends chose their obstetrician or midwife on the recommendation of other friends or their own GP. But this decision is very personal. I have another friend who wanted a female obstetrician. She said that having a male obstetrician was like having a vegetarian teach you how to barbecue ribs.

It is vital that your wife likes the obstetrician and feels comfortable with him or her. It is also important that you both find out the doctor's attitudes and practices towards intervention, pain relief, birth positions, C-sections, the role of the father and so on. You don't want to discover in the delivery room that your ideas and expectations are vastly different.

Hospital or Home?

Even today, "home births" are the norm for millions of women around the world. While not too many Western women take up this option, many would say that a midwife-assisted home birth is still a reasonable choice for a healthy woman who has had an uncomplicated pregnancy and is within reach of medical services should they be required.

Some couples find hospitals impersonal and disempowering, so they opt for having their babies at home. It is perhaps more comfortable and relaxed to give birth in familiar surroundings, and, although the birth is supervised by a midwife, there is minimal medical intervention. It also allows more flexibility in terms of having a water birth or having family and friends assisting in particular ways. Some couples choose home birth because it means their older children or friends can be present – which, ironically, is exactly the same reason why other couples choose *not* to have a home birth.

Home births account for just over 1 percent of all births in America, and it looks like that figure will stay pretty small in the future. Some health-insurance companies do not cover home births, so you may have to pay the midwife's fees yourself, making it more expensive than a hospital birth. In addition, recent changes in the world of liability insurance mean that it is difficult (read: "next to impossible") for midwives to get insurance to cover themselves. And, for fear of getting sued, fewer midwives are willing to put their necks on the line. The American Congress of Obstetricians and Gynecologists believes hospitals and birth centers are the safest settings for birth but respects a woman's right to make this decision.

We decided against a home birth for three reasons:

1. We didn't like the possibility of neighbors dropping in for a cup of tea in the middle of it all.
2. The whole idea scared me to death. We wanted the resources of a fully equipped multibillion-dollar hospital, complete with expert personnel and expensive machines and a doctor who had done it thousands of times before and had lots of impressive certificates hanging on his or her surgery wall.
3. New carpets in the house. Say no more.

Other couples (two percent) opt for birth centers, which are more "homey" and low-tech than hospitals. These centers have a more relaxed atmosphere, a less sterile decor and an ethos of non-interventionist birthing methods. They are run by midwives and often are a separate unit of a hospital so staff have access to additional medical support if necessary.

The majority of birthing women still go to a hospital. Ideally, your hospital should be near your home, so you can reach it relatively quickly without having to run red lights or drive on sidewalks like they do in the movies. The most fantastic hospital in the world is no good if it is on the other side of the city. If you get stuck in a traffic jam, you might even run the risk of having the baby in the back of the car, which will lower its resale value significantly.

Public or Private?

If you elect for your baby to be born in a hospital, your next choice will be whether to go public or private. Part of this choice will be dictated by your health cover. Make no mistake: while it doesn't have to be, childbirth can be expensive. All you have to do is look at what's parked in the "Reserved for Doctors Only" car spaces at the hospital to realize that there is a lot of money involved in this whole childbirth thing.

After you or your wife has phoned up the hospital to make the booking, your wife will probably have to go in for a meeting, fill out forms giving personal details and generally answer a lot of questions. The hospital will also want to know what kind of health coverage she has, if any.

Your wife can go to your local *public hospital* as a *public patient*, which means she gets the specialist who is on duty in the hospital at the time. As the name suggests, the facilities are public. The women there may have to share rooms and bathrooms (although several of my friends have countered this with experiences where they paid $0 and had great care and great facilities with no room sharing. Then again, while they say they paid $0, the car-park fees made up for it). I have friends who wouldn't go anywhere but the local public hospital and others who are the exact opposite. It depends on your financial situation and your expectations. Going public is the least expensive option, particularly if you have no insurance. Check out your local hospital and see what you think. Ask around about its reputation in the local community.

If you want to go private, you have a choice. Selecting a hospital is like most things: you need to shop around to make an informed decision about what's best for you. Most hospitals have a labor-ward tour you can go on so you can fully check out the facilities. (One of my friends who went private chose the "platinum package," which included wine and meals for dad and a large double room so he could stay there as well.) Ask your friends for recommendations, talk to your family doctor and visit some hospitals. You'll also find internet forums and blogs a rich source of commentary about various hospitals and people's experiences of them. Having said that, trying to juggle strings of essentially opposite and contradictory online opinions can be an exercise in futility and frustration, much like trying to make sense of user reviews of hotels, restaurants, movies or books.

It is important to have a very clear understanding of what is covered by your health insurance. The best thing is to get on the phone to your insurance company or visit their website. Maternity care and childbirth are covered as essential health benefits, so you can get coverage even if you were pregnant before getting insurance. Be famililar with the terms of your plan. Check the fine print in relation to what is covered by way of public/private hospitals. Also bear in mind that your wife's insurance might cover the baby for the first 30 days of its life, but it depends on the policy, so you need to take steps to ensure your newborn baby will also be covered. This will likely involve upgrading to some sort of family policy, which will cover your baby in the case of any unforeseen issues arising that could require intervention or specialist or extended care.

For the birth of Rachael, Meredith had private insurance and went as a *private patient* to our local *public hospital*. This meant that, because we had the insurance, we could afford Meredith's own obstetrician (see previous). But we wanted the local public hospital because it was closest to our home and we were familiar with it, since we had been to birth classes there. The maternity ward also had a solid reputation and the staff were great. The hospital had a warm and welcoming atmosphere, and it just felt right.

However, there were some things about the hospital that we weren't too happy about afterwards. During the first stage of labor, Meredith had to share one bathroom with three other laboring women who were in equal need of the facility. We were all in the same large room and the curtains did little to shield us from their collective wailing and moaning. After the birth, the visiting hours were not strictly enforced, so Meredith was bombarded by guests almost all day and got tired very quickly. She also shared a room with a woman who was always visited by at least ten relatives with very loud voices. To top it off, this woman had a baby who screamed *non-stop*. It is good to know, however, that things have changed. Several of our new-parent friends utilized their local public hospitals, and cannot speak highly enough of the facilities and the staff and the experience.

For the births of Georgia and Matilda, Meredith went as a *private patient* to a *private hospital*. We were both more confident the second and third time around and so were happy about travelling a greater distance to reach this hospital. Meredith had her own room, so she got some peace and quiet, and her own en suite, which made life a bit easier. The staff were ever-vigilant about visiting hours, too. Dads could visit anytime, but if you weren't a dad and you arrived out of visiting hours, you'd never make it past the nurses, who patrolled the corridors packing cattle prods. In terms of cost, all up with our private insurance the gap was just several hundred dollars. If it wasn't for the insurance, however, the births would have set us back several thousand. But that's what you pay for a maternity ward that serves king prawns and lava cake for dinner.

A final word of warning, however: if you decide to go to a private hospital, you will need to book in quickly. Spaces are limited and they go faster than Super Bowl tickets.

Some questions you might like to consider when choosing a hospital are:

- What is the availability of toilets and showers?
- What are the rooms like?
- Do they have facilities for "different" types of births, or do they stick to "traditional" methods?
- What are their statistics regarding Caesarean interventions (which is obviously connected to the obstetricians frequenting that hospital).
- What is their attitude toward pain relief?
- How long do they let mothers stay to recover after the birth?

- Is there a patient rest period each day when visitors aren't allowed in?
- What magazines do they have in the kiosk?
- How good is the coffee in their cafe?
- Do they have a nearby emergency ward, in case a father faints and splits his head open on the concrete floor and has to be taken away for stitches?

Whatever decisions you make, you probably want to get onto it sooner rather than later. Another thing you need to find out is how much you will be charged. This is *very important*. European luxury cars are expensive to run, and the money comes from one place. That's right – *you*. Once again, you should check your insurance coverage.

Check-Ups and Monitoring

It is the midwife or obstetrician's job to monitor both mother and baby during the pregnancy and then to be there to supervise the birth and "deliver" the baby. Part of this monitoring process involves a series of check-ups. These take place monthly but can be every two weeks as the birth draws closer, and then every week. During these visits, your wife's blood, urine, weight and blood pressure are tested. These visits also test your wife's patience, as invariably she will sit for three hours waiting for her appointment.

On several occasions, I was able to go along with Meredith to her check-ups. I found this to be really beneficial, because I got to meet and know the obstetrician and was able to ask all the questions that were flooding my mind ("What happens if the baby is too big to get out?," "What happens if the contractions start too early?," "How's the fuel consumption of your new Audi?"). This was also a great way to share the experience of pregnancy and helped me to prepare for what lay ahead.

On one of these occasions, the obstetrician put a microphoney thing (a fetal stethoscope) on Meredith's pregnant bit and we sat in awe, listening to the gallop of our unborn baby's heart. This was a great thrill! It really made me realize that there was a little person in there. If you can, be there to experience this.

Another thing the obstetrician does is calculate the expected date of birth. A normal pregnancy lasts, as you know, about nine months, although it is "normal" for babies to be born between thirty-seven and forty-two weeks. However, the baby doesn't have a calendar in the womb and might not want to wait until the conveniently predicted ninth month to tick over before deciding to make the grand entrance. Premature babies can be born from seven months, or twenty-eight weeks, into the pregnancy, although obviously, the more premature it is, the less developed it is and the likelihood of complications increases significantly.

Personally, I wonder if this whole "due date" thing is a bit of a professional conspiracy among obstetricians. I can almost picture it. Many years ago, at the Annual Conference for Obstetricians with Flashy Cars, one leant across to some others and said, "Hey, guys, I've got this really great joke that we can all play on nervous expectant couples . . ."

Thanks to the German obstetrician F. K. Naegele (who devised this method almost 200 years ago), due dates are calculated by counting forward nine months from the female's last menstrual period (yes, using your fingers is okay) and adding seven days, but I suspect it's done with a dart thrown onto a calendar. The doctor may also ask your wife to have an ultrasound to confirm the due date, as well as to check out a few other things.

There is no doubt that we live in a wonderful age of technology. We have at our disposal all sorts of fantastic gizmos, apps and whirligigs that can do all sorts of amazing and incredible things that our parents would never have believed possible. Sure, some of our advancements have been a big mistake and have only served to drag humanity down further into the abyss of self-destruction (cloning, the Tiddy Bear [LMGTFY], beauty pageants for children, social media, paraphilic infantilism, reality TV, the Snuggie, etc.). But some of the advancements seem to have generally been quite a good idea, and make our lives a lot better (smartphone, Velcro, the Leatherman tool, guitars with in-built tuners, the Snuggie, etc.) and one of the best is the ultrasound. Since the dawn of time, mom and dad have had to wait for the grand debut, the moment of birth, to get their first look at junior. These days are long gone, thanks to the marvels of modern medical technology.

Here's how the ultrasound works. You and your wife go down to the local radiology clinic, there to sit in the waiting room reading about "My Miracle Octuplets" in a well-thumbed *Reader's Digest*. At some point exasperatingly after the time you thought it was going to happen, you are called in to get on the table (wife, not you). The radiographer comes in and probes the swollen front bit of your wife (where the baby lives) with a microphone probe (technically, a transducer). This sends out high-frequency soundwaves (hence *ultra*-sound), which are then reflected back and processed onto a monitor for you all to see.

And there you have it.

Your child.

The radiographer will say amazing things to you such as "There's baby's arm," "There's baby's head" and "Baby's facing *this* way."

There were moments during each of Meredith's pregnancies where I wondered if this whole ultrasound thing was a prank. It always looked to me like Meredith was giving birth to a satellite photo of Earth. There were our baby's legs (cumulus clouds over Sydney), her chest (low-pressure front moving north), and her head (cyclone off the coast). But who wants to be the first one to ask "Sorry, are we just looking at a badly tuned TV station?," so instead I found myself excitedly coming out with "Hey, yeah, wow . . . I think I see . . . a hand." *Liar!*

More recent technology has improved things considerably in the form of rendered 3D images or 4D imaging video. These 3D/4D gold-colored images are kind of spooky – looking a bit like death masks you find in old penal museums – but they are a breathtaking insight into what is happening in the womb.

The other exciting thing about a visit to the radiographer is that not only do you get to see the image on the screen, but you can take home some souvenirs as well. For starters, you can get snapshot "photos" of the scan. These look like X-rays, with body-part labels so you can identify exactly what it is you are looking at (jellyfish = head, bacon = forearm, coathanger = pelvis, snowflakes = skin, etc.) You can start your own baby-photo album months before the birth, and there's nothing like a good ultrasound snap to excite your Facebook "friends" or get a YouTube vibe going. Or you can take home a thumb drive with the rendered ultrasound video, allowing you to relive it in real time in the comfort of your own home. Definitely a keeper for your son/daughter's twenty-first birthday party.

I'm sure it won't be long before radiographers really grasp the true potential of ultrasound marketing and start producing stuff like ultrasound print T-shirts, or those plastic domes with a replica fetus inside. All you do is shake . . . and it snows!

An ultrasound achieves four things.

First, as already mentioned, it can confirm the estimated "due date." This is done by measuring the length of one of the baby's bones. Invariably, the due date is quite different to the one supplied to you originally. (And simply adds weight to my previously mentioned theory regarding "due dates.")

Second, it checks and confirms that everything is okay and all the baby's bits are where they're supposed to be.

Third, you can tell how many babies are in there. Odds are that it is only going to be one. But if you can count four legs, either your wife is going to give birth to a horse or you're going to be the parents of twins.

The only somewhat reliable Hellin's Law dictates that you have about a one in eighty-nine chance of having twins, a one in eighty-nine^2 chance of having triplets, a one in eighty-nine^3 chance of having quadruplets (and so on). If you can count seven or more pairs of legs, sell your car and buy a minibus. (And just be thankful that you aren't Feodor Vassilyev, a Russian whose wife, in a world-record feat of reproduction, gave birth to sixteen pairs of twins, seven sets of triplets and four sets of quadruplets – sixty-nine children in all. Actually, no. Just be thankful you aren't Mrs. Vassilyeva.)

Fourth, in addition to all the medical reassurances and information that come from an ultrasound, there is some-thing momentous about seeing and hearing the pulsing heart of your child – a rapid *buda-buda-buda-buda* beat like a tense sonar moment in a WW2 submarine movie – that makes it all seem more real, as you see and hear that there really is a little person in there.

And . . . ready or not . . . you're going to be a dad.

Life's Little Changes

When your wife is pregnant, stuff starts to . . . *change*.

These changes may be subtle at first, but as the months inexorably tick by, things will start to seem "different." You will notice that your wife is beginning to . . . *transform*.

There are hormonal changes. Her body is super-charged with progesterone and estrogen, and so you may cop mood swings as unpredictable as the weather that time you ill-advisedly booked a beach trip during hurricane season. For example, in answer to the question "Would you like some tea?" you could get a simple "Yes, please" or "No, thanks." However, you could also get a teary "That's the most beautiful thing you've ever said to me" or an aggressive "Don't *patronize* me! I can make my own tea!"

While most pregnant women won't fit the weepy or cranky stereotype bandied about on television sitcoms (or in the paragraph above), it is understandably not uncommon for them to take a ride on the mood roller-coaster. Other side effects on the pregnancy smorgasbord may include cravings, headaches, clumsiness, heartburn, fluid retention, high blood pressure, cramps, vagueness, anxiety, irrational decision-making and tiredness.

And there's still the aforementioned morning sickness. What can you do to help? I've heard of different remedies, such as dry toast, back rubs, glucose, ginger, steam inhalation, frequent small meals, lots of fluids, herbal tea and a clove of garlic hung around the neck. Some people swear by iron tablets or saline drips, and there's one remedy involving a cat, a battery and a tube of toothpaste, but the less said about that, the better.

Morning sickness will happen when it wants to and you can't stop it. However, you can help not to make it worse than it already is. Make your wife a cup of tea before she gets out of bed. Don't bait your fishing line in front of her. When cooking, avoid fatty and spicy foods, and strong or aromatic herbs. Most importantly, if she looks green, don't stand between her and the bathroom. Be supportive and undemanding, allowing her to do whatever she needs to in order to cope with nausea.

One increasingly obvious change is that your wife is getting bigger, because the baby is getting bigger, but that means that all her other internal bits and pieces have less and less room (#decreasedbladder). In short, it means that your own lengthy interludes in the bathroom with the latest *Phantom* comic or new-fave phone app will have to be cut short. It also means that epic road trips may need to be rethought. Don't mess with a woman with a bladder the size of a walnut.

Overall, your wife will gain around 25 to 35 pounds. Interestingly, only about a third of this gain is the weight of the baby. The other weight is made up of the placenta and increases in blood, amniotic fluid, fat and the uterus. The most obvious sign of this gain is that your wife won't be able to fit into those old denim jeans or her favorite dress anymore. Coincidentally, it's around this time that you notice a lot of your own clothes go missing, particularly big and baggy sweaters, T-shirts and jerseys. On top of this, she will probably need to break out the credit card and go buying a new range of fashion tents, also referred to as "maternity wear."

Another obvious change is the increase in the size of your wife's breasts. This kicks in around the three-month mark. The change is caused by the mammary glands in her breasts getting ready for all the important and hard work ahead of them in feeding a child. The breasts will get bigger and the nipples and areolae larger and darker. Within the areolae, the little glands or bumps surrounding the nipples will become more pronounced. (Curiously, these are called the Glands of Montgomery, apparently after an Irish doctor who wrote about them in the 1800s. Personally, I think this is a rather inflated and grandiose title, giving rise to ridiculous images of an Arctic-type explorer standing atop a giant breast and stabbing it with a flag, declaring in a haughty accent, "In the name of King and Country, I declare these . . . the Glands of Montgomery!') But although your wife's breasts are swollen and impressive, they are probably quite sore. While you might be boggle-eyed in the presence of her invitingly engorged bosom, do not misconstrue this as license to grope; i.e., keep your damn hands to yourself.

While these physical changes can make life awkward, they are not always as paralizing as television moms would have us believe. (See Chapter One.) Pregnancy and child-birth are normal and healthy. A pregnant woman is not "sick" and shouldn't be treated as such. Having said that, your wife certainly won't be as nimble as she used to be. Due to the new weight distribution, she may have a sore back or legs. Many everyday activities can become increasingly awkward and even painful for her. Sleeping becomes quite uncomfort-able as, in addition to the less than convenient new shape of her body, she may have to cope with such troublesome maladies as heartburn, increased heart rate, shortness of breath and a frequent need to go to the toilet. In fact, towards the end of the pregnancy, nearly all sleeping positions can be quite uncomfortable, so do all you can to help out. Stuff pillows in all the right places for support. There is an extensive range of full-body pillows, maternity pillows and pillow wedges available on the market, although you can probably achieve the same result with a spare blanket and some loose cushions.

While you shouldn't treat her as though she's a porcelain doll, there are plenty of other things you can do to make your wife's life a little easier as her pregnancy progresses. Do more than your "fair share" of the shopping, cooking, cleaning, washing and ironing. Give her back rubs on demand. Provide breakfast in bed. Be understanding if her aching body or nausea means rearranging social engagements, including your planned holiday hiking in Yellowstone.

More on Sex

Ah, yes – this is what caused all this fuss in the first place. *And you want more?*

Sex is a normal and healthy thing for a couple who love each other. And sex is possible and normal during pregnancy.

Having said that, you have to use your common sense. The female body goes through incredible changes during pregnancy. Because one of these is hormonal, you may find that your wife's previously voracious sexual appetite has dimmed somewhat. In short, she may not "feel like it." It may not be as frequent as "before." In these circumstances, it can be easy for husbands to feel resentful or cranky that things have changed, even some level of hurt that your wife doesn't "want" you. These feelings are normal and okay. It is important that you come to terms with this and bear in mind all the massive hormonal and physical changes with which her body is trying to cope. If you need some sensitivity training in this area, get yourself a whopper hangover, strap a beanbag and a couple of house bricks around your stomach and then see how you feel about sex.

And even when you do engage in sex or sexual play, there are physical limitations. You will find that it's not as acrobatic or convenient as it once might have been (i.e., swinging from light fixtures, wholesale destruction of bedroom furniture, anything *Kama Sutra* or drinking pina coladas and making love at midnight in the dunes of the Cape). You will need to be a little more creative in terms of getting the pieces of the puzzle to fit together comfortably, if you get my drift. Try some different positions and even different furniture for support.

Of course, all women are different. It's important that the two of you discuss your sexuality together. It's important that you are understanding and respectful and supportive of her. Sex is a good and normal part of relationships, but pregnancy can temporarily alter the normal pattern. This is not a permanent state. Down the track, things get back to normal. Oh yes, they do. Trust me. Oh yes.

And, by the way, if you think your pregnant wife is off-limits because your whopping great fertility organ will be a physical threat to the baby, *don't flatter yourself.*

Of Opossums and Men

I feel sorry for the male opossum. There he is, enjoying *coitus opossumatus* in a comfortable branch of his favorite tree, when only thirteen days later – that's right, count 'em – his mate gives birth to an opossumette. This probably accounts for the low life expectancy of male opossums.

Luckily, we non-marsupials have a little more leeway. Nine months is quite a decent period in which to get ready for our new station in life. But this does not mean that parents-to-be have nine months to relax and party on. Use this valuable time to work hard in preparing for the arrival of your human-ette. And, believe me, it *is* hard work. Spend your time wisely. (See Chapter Three.)

Don't be fooled into thinking that this time will go slowly. We're not as fortunate as the African elephant, which has a gestation period of about twenty-one months. African-elephant dads certainly have no excuse if *they're* not ready for life on the plains with a young pachyderm.

As I mentioned earlier, it's common in the early stages of their wife's pregnancy for dads-to-be to feel a bit disori-entated. Already, everyone who knows you're going to be a dad has started treating you differently, your sex life has an "Endangered Species" stamp on it, you've nobly stood by your wife in steering clear of gin and tonics, you've stared in dismay at your bank balance, your wife has vomited in the bathroom – and it's only been twenty-four hours since you heard the news.

Welcome to pregnancy.

But don't worry. Unlike the opossum, you still have several months to get ready.

3

Brace Yourself

"When the nesting urge comes, don't fight it.
You'll only make things worse."

Facing the Facts

Okay, let's get straight into it: life as you have known it is over.

Finito. Ende. Kaput. Sayonara. Hasta la vista, baby.

So long. Farewell. *Auf Wiedersehen*. Goodbye.

Gone. History. Jurassic.

Pregnancy is an Extinction Level Event.

The sooner you get used to this, the better.

Your life as a dad will be totally different from anything you have previously known. It sure changed my life. It may come as a surprise to you, but I didn't always drive a minivan filled with car seats and boosters and popcorn, and I never used to leave parties at 10 pm. I haven't always hung out at the wading pool at the local swim center. My idea of a great night hasn't always been fish sticks and string cheese in front of the latest Pixar movie. And those stains on my shirts didn't used to be there.

But that was *before*.

Get used to the fact that you can't be a CWOC (couple with one child) or a CASK (couple and several kids) while trying to live like a DINK (double income, no kids) or a SINK (single income, no kids). The lifestyles, responsibilities, roles and daily routines of CWOCs, CASKs, DINKs and SINKs are totally different, opposed and mutually exclusive. If you try to live like a DINK when you're a CWOC, you will find it frustrating and exhausting. And trying to live like a SINK when you're a CASK is impossible. You'll end up wishing you were still a WANKA (without any new kids anyway).

What I'm talking about is your use of time. You used to have a lot of it to throw around and please yourself with. Game of golf this afternoon? *Sure!* Beer after work? *Yes!* Knock off another novel in the hammock? *Great!* An impromptu movie? *Certainly!* A weekend surf safari? *Why not?* House renovations? *Nothing better to do!*

But not anymore. The responsibility of active fathering demands your time. Parenting takes time. Your child needs your time. (Getting the point?) There are no short cuts or ways around this.

There are three main areas in which you'll need to deliberately do some basic time management over the next twelve months.

First, there are the *coming months of pregnancy*. You and your wife will be busy getting ready for the arrival of a new person in your home. This is an especially time-consuming operation, involving a pretty robust list of "things to do." But the better you prepare now, the better it will be for you later on.

Second, there is the expected time of arrival, often referred to as the *due date* or *mission improbable*. You need to attack your calendars and devices and diaries – both home and work – in the weeks surrounding this elusive date, since babies don't usually follow adult timetables. It is extremely important that you are available and on call when that giant roulette wheel in the sky drops the ball and your baby arrives. And you need to be around in the weeks that follow. This is a tumultuous time, when a heavy work and/or social schedule will not help the situation.

As an employee, you have certain rights around taking leave when your child is born. Check your work contract and the Family and Medical Leave Act (FMLA) website to find out what you are eligible for by way of unpaid and paid parental leave. Give your employer the heads up about the due date and talk about what it means for you to disappear at zero notice. If your work allows you any flexibility, avoid loading up the weeks around the due date. (Don't book overseas trips, golf days, conferences or expensive theater seats around this time either.) A lot of my friends took their paternity leave or vacation time so they could be around during those crucial first weeks at home. But be careful: just because you high-lighted a day in your calendar doesn't mean the baby is going to come then. It could be weeks before or after.

And third, in the longer term (and by *longer term* I mean, say, the next twenty years), your *new family life* will be time-consuming. Coming home from work at ridiculous hours, commitments on every weekend and weeknight (training, school, gigs, gym, movies, rehearsals, pub nights, visiting buddies, late meetings, concerts, games, sitting on your ass betting on the horses, etc.), and raging on weekends until the wee hours will leave you with very little time to be a father (or a husband, for that matter). Essentially, while there will, in truth, still be time for "you," there will be less than before, because being a dad means that you have to – and will want to – share that with others; namely, your family.

You have probably come across the expression "quality time." The theory behind this is that you spend intensive time with your child, focused on them, rather than having them in your vicinity while you read the paper or update your status. This could be cuddling them, singing to them, taking them for a walk, talking to them. Such "quality time" is important, as long as it is not misused. You cannot make up for working ridiculous hours and never being at home by grabbing a desperate thirty minutes of book reading once every blue moon.

Instead, you also need to think in terms of "quantity time." This is simply the very mundane domestic act of hanging around the house and spending time with your family doing everyday stuff. In short, your child simply needs you to "be around." I'm not suggesting that you leave your job and enter some la-la dad fantasy rainbow world where you spend twenty-four hours a day with your family. Obviously, there'll be times when things are hectic and work demands much of your attention. In some ways, it is an unavoidable part of our contemporary work ethic. But, as a general rule, your family gets priority.

So sit down with your wife and talk over your weekly schedules. Basically, once the baby comes, you'll want to spend a lot of time at home. This won't happen magically of its own accord. It takes deliberate thought and effort on your part to establish new divisions of labor and time, and it just might mean you'll have to toss some things in.

It all sounds pretty bleak, doesn't it? Well, it's not. It's just different.

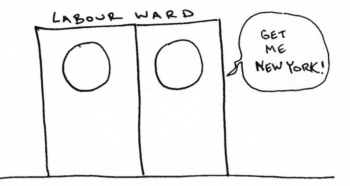

At first, you'll still be able to operate pretty much as normal. Newborns are portable and generally sedate, so you can take them with you to dinner parties or soccer matches without too much hassle. Later, when they're older and outings become more difficult, you and your wife can work as a team and take turns in looking after the baby while the other goes out. Things such as sports, part-time study, social gatherings, rehearsals, club meetings and so on can all be juggled in moderation. In fact, it is healthy for you and your wife to find and plan some spaces in your schedule where you can just each have some down time to yourself to do whatever (go for a walk, restring your guitar, grab a coffee, surf, trim a hedge . . .). Babysitters, relatives and baby-crazy friends can also give you the opportunity to go out together.

Sure, you lose some freedom. But there are no freebies in this world, and that's part of the new deal of the privilege and pleasure of being a dad.

By the way, when I said that it's not really that bleak, I was kidding.

Working in a Coalmine

Some jobs are just plain hard to do when there's another person living and growing inside your own body space. If your wife is a judo instructor, for example, she will find it increasingly difficult to fulfill her work commitments. Also, she may find it hard if she works in a place where she is on her feet all day or has to lift weighty things or go up lots of stairs or ladders or deal with chemicals or radiation. As the pregnancy progresses, she will tend to get tired more quickly. Aching muscles will come with increasing regularity. Eventually, there will come a time when work will have to go. Most bosses don't want their employees having babies while on company grounds; carpet shampoo is expensive.

When Meredith was pregnant with Rachael, she was working for a government department on the other side of the city. That meant a considerable peak-hour bus journey every morning, followed by another bus journey and then a good walk before she reached her workplace. As the weeks went by, getting to work became more challenging. Not only was there the daily terror of a potential vomiting-on-a-crowded-bus scenario but also, in the early stages of her pregnancy, she often found herself standing uncomfortably for long periods.

I optimistically attribute this lack of chivalry on the part of nearby seated guys to being stuck in that awkward public-transport middle ground between wanting to do the right thing (pregnant lady needing a seat?), but maybe not being quite sure that she *is* actually pregnant (*not* pregnant lady with slight paunch about to take offense at your suggestion that she needs a seat?). Thanks, feminism. I cling to the hope that obviously pregnant women on buses still get offered a seat.

Meredith fronted the challenges of work and the difficulties of public transport for several months before deciding that enough was enough. However, there is no set time for when a pregnant woman has to leave work. It's up to how she feels, although I suspect that the dark shadow of mortgage repayments puts a heavy strain on many couples these days. Some women enjoy the luxury of being able to leave work as soon as they "hear the news." Others, for reasons of finance or job commitment or sanity, stick it out for as long as they can.

The choices regarding leaving work are not extensive. Women can either leave their positions for good or they can take maternity leave. There are a range of maternity-leave regulations and variations in place, so your wife should consult her relevant personnel department, union or industry body for the specifics that apply to her situation. The Family and Medical Leave Act website also outlines current regulations. (While it is illegal to discriminate in the workplace against a pregnant woman, there may be specific limitations in relation to her job, for example if she works with hazardous substances or is a commercial pilot, police officer or air-traffic controller.)

You and your wife should also discuss work arrangements for after the birth. You can't just leave a newborn in its crib for the day while you both go off to work. Someone has to look after the baby. How you resolve this issue will be influenced by a number of factors, such as: your attitudes towards your jobs and/or careers; how flexible your workplaces are; how big your mortgage repayments are; which of you earns the most money; your attitudes to breast- and/or bottle-feeding; how you feel about daycare; how much cash you have in the bank; the willingness and capability of well-meaning nearby grandparents who are itching to get in on some serious grandparent time; and which of you has the stronger will.

There are all sorts of possibilities and solutions open to you. Meredith and I had a fairly traditional approach. Despite having a university degree and a career path, Meredith decided to leave work to take up the position of Mother and Domestic Manager with a new but rapidly growing business called The Downey Family. Doing it this way isn't so hot financially, but it does make for a secure and consistent home environment, which we both value.

There are many other approaches available to you, depending on how flexible or innovative you want to be. The couple across the road from us take turns in working and being at home for periods of roughly one year, thus giving each of them an experience of life as a full-time parent. Of course, it doesn't make for a smooth climb up the career ladder. I also once met a couple who worked out their jobs so that they both got to experience full-time parenting and full-time work. The mom worked the day shift (8 am until 4 pm) and the dad worked the night shift (3 pm until 11 pm). The baby was minded for two hours in the interim. It was good for them financially, but the problem was that they only saw each other as husband and wife late at night or on Sundays. This was not particularly conducive to the development of a marriage.

Other friends I know both hold down nine-to-five jobs while the baby's grandparents play babysitters during the day. The service is free and the grandparents relish the opportunity to spend time with their grandchild. Not everybody has this opportunity at their disposal, though. Similarly, privately employing the services of a nanny or au pair can give good in-home continuity, but you'd better be really wealthy.

Certain organizations and licensed individuals also run family daycare and daycare centers.

Family daycare ("home-based care") is where your baby is minded in the carer's (or educator's) home. It provides a stable environment for your baby, with close supervision from the carer. In most states, official family day cares have to be licensed and meet certain regulations; however, in some states centers are license-exempt, so be familiar with the requirements in your area. As a relatively low-cost service, family child care homes are a very popular choice for working couples.

Other childcare centers ("long daycare") are larger, sometimes caring for up to forty children at a time. The advantage of these centers is that, unlike in the family-daycare situation, if the regular carer is sick, there is still someone else available to look after your baby. Often, your baby can be minded for longer hours, too. There are only two drawbacks: it's often difficult to get a place for your baby, and you have to pay more for it. Waiting lists for little babies can be up to eighteen months long, because babies are more labor-intensive than your average semi-independent toddler. Babies can also be more expensive. Some private daycare centers could cost you hundreds each week, depending on the number of hours your baby spends there.

The thing to do is to put your baby's name (if it *has* a name, but more about that later) down on the lists of childcare places *as soon as possible.* No matter where you decide to go, check it out. Each state's set standards for licensing daycare centers are different, but they are readily available on the internet. If you're given a place, go down and check out the facilities and the carers. You will very soon get a feel for the center. If, for example, the carer in charge is wearing an "Anarchy Forever" T-shirt, you might want to try somewhere else.

If your wife does decide to go back to the paid workforce – in whatever capacity – she probably won't be doing it straight away. I mean, there's nothing stopping her from going back the day after the baby is born, if she really wants to – that is, assuming she can still walk. However, most women returning to the workforce go back usually around three to six months after the birth. By then, they can walk without hobbling, their breastmilk doesn't soak their blouses and people have stopped asking them "When are you due?"

Nesting Urge

In the period immediately before they reproduce, most birds and mammals experience what is commonly known as the nesting urge. This is an instinct whereby the female goes into a frenzy of preparing a safe space for their newborn to live. Rabbits dig a burrow. Birds build a nest. Cats find a dark corner in the garage.

Pregnant women also get the nesting urge.

Now, although your wife hopefully won't be up a tree making a little basket out of twigs, cotton, mud and saliva, the nesting urge will definitely manifest itself in its own cute way. It is unavoidable. It's a hormonal thing. In women's brains, just under the hypothalamus, there is a small gland that secretes nesting-urge hormone. When this gland starts operating, you will notice some changes in your wife . . . such as an absence of logic, no concept of reason, a demand for exceptional tidiness and a strong desire to make major architectural changes to your home.

As a young married couple, we were fortunate to be able to live in my old family home. We decided to make a room for the baby in my old bedroom, which remained as a fire-engine-red "den," complete with low mood lighting and decorations on the wall (such as old car license plates). Yeah, I know. Cool. All the furniture was built-in and connected at different levels: bed, cupboards, bookshelves, drawers and a desk. The crowning glory was a huge, pool-hall-style, rice-paper lampshade, complete with tassels, which dangled from the ceiling.

A perfect room for a baby!

So I thought.

I remember the day clearly. Returning from work, I pulled into the driveway and immediately knew something was awry. This was primarily because of the large mountain of red splintered wood in the middle of the backyard which strangely reminded me of my old bedroom furniture.

In a daze, I made my way into the house, clambering over an enormous roll of shredded carpet that I'm pretty sure wasn't there when I'd left for work that morning. In the shell of my old room, I found my excessively pregnant wife, bathed in sweat and grime, blithely chiselling sheets of old paint and wallpaper and license plates off the walls. Half the room was already stripped back to bare, grey concrete. I stood there for a while, mouth agape, before I spoke.

"What are you doing?" I asked carefully, so as not to startle her.

"Making a nursery."

"Oh."

"I thought a nice yellow would do. We can sand back the picture rails so they'll match the floorboards. Of course, we'll have to sand those back too."

"Mmm," I said, slowly backing out of the room, being careful not to break eye contact.

At that point, I felt a migraine coming on, so I bailed and poured myself a bourbon.

When the nesting urge comes, don't fight it. You'll only make things worse.

Digital Parenting

Another sea you will have to navigate on your journey into fatherhood is the mighty internet. Tim Berners-Lee's invention has turned out to be both a blessing and a curse. On the one hand, it has so much to offer new parents. But there are also many hazards and pitfalls, and it is important you go in with your eyes open before typing into Google, "Which stroller is the best?"

So let's unpack what it means to be a dad (and mom) in a digital age, looking at some of the advantages and disadvantages.

Advantages

Access to Information

Throughout human history, dads haven't really needed to know too much about fetal development, or the mystery of childbirth, or anything else to do with being a dad.

That's changed in the last few generations, with dads now expected (and wanting) to be more involved. Up till recently, though, the information at their disposal was pretty limited. You could look something up in an encyclopaedia (P is for Pregnancy), borrow a book from a library (*DIY Crib*!), do a course ("Breathe . . . breathe . . ."), or maybe find a brochure at the hospital ("Why Does My Baby Cry All the Time?").

The internet's changed all that, and never before have dads had so much information at their literal fingertips about anything and everything to do with being a dad. Whether it's comparing Diaper Brand A to Diaper Brand B or finding out what an episiotomy is; whether it's price-comparing car seats or watching footage of real babies being born; whether it's checking out hospitals or needing travel-crib-assembly instructions; whether it's knowing the difference between a Naegele scan and an Apgar test . . . if you want it, there are millions of places for you to go: websites, news articles, animations, pictures, forums, videos, press releases, blogs, online communities, research papers, government reports, fact sheets, statistics, charts. Yep, the internet has put dad in the proverbial parenting-info candy shop.

Sharing

One of the cool things about being a dad is sharing your journey with your friends and family. This is, after all, a special and momentous time in your life. They'll be excited by your "pregnancy news," watching carefully how things are going through the pregnancy, waiting eagerly for the "big day" (Boy or girl? Name? Weight? Yay!), and then wanting to meet and get to know your newest family member as they grow up.

This used to be a labor-intensive exercise. There were individual phone calls and visits and letters to announce the pregnancy. The birth was generally proclaimed to the world in a painstaking sequence via the payphone in the maternity-ward lobby and in the following days to everyone in your phone book; or, further afield, by methodically producing a run of handwritten letters (featuring, for parents with a creative flair, a baby foot or hand paint imprint), complete with addressing envelopes, licking stamps and posting them to all and sundry. And, if your friends or family wanted to see how the little tyke was going in the coming months, they had to turn up at your house with a coffee cake on a Sunday afternoon.

The internet has simplified things considerably. An ever-growing panoply of social-media options now allows you to broadcast your dadhood and baby news to the world in real time. Click a photo, tap out a few words ("Pregnant wife!," "Baby born!," "Baby yawning!," "Selfie of Dad changing diaper!"), press send . . . done. You can connect with whomever you want, whenever you want, wherever you are with one hand, while making Eggs Benedict with the other. It is convenient and fast and has the added benefit that you can manipulate your status/photos/updates/tweets to maximize how cool you look, how amah-zing your baby is and what an easy and fun time you are having being a new dad. Sweet! (Take *that*, ex-girlfriend! Not so much of a loser now, hey?)

Community and Support

Some new dads seem to have an intuitive sense and confidence about what to do with babies and how to be a dad. I was not one of those guys. I was anxious, cautious and uncertain on many levels. It's not that I was stupid or uninterested or anything. I was just *out of my depth*.

There may be times during your wife's pregnancy or your early dad days when you are concerned and uncertain about something and feel kind of weird and alone, and maybe even embarrassed to raise your darkest doubts. As social beings, we crave to know that we are not alone, that all is okay, that I am not the first dad on the planet to live through this, and that what I am going through is, well, *normal*. In fact, it seems to me from my digital perusing that one of the most common questions asked in dad/parent forums is "Is this normal?":

- My wife isn't so interested in sex anymore. Is this normal?
- My baby wakes up four times a night. Is this normal?

- I'm so bloody tired. Is this normal?
- My wife's nipples are blue. Is this normal?
- My baby seems to poop out more than its own body weight. Is this normal?
- The travel-crib instructions say I have to lift up the para-pluie rib assembly until the locking pins click into the vertical struts, but only once all seven Velcro tabs have been released and I hand-tighten the reticulated nuts . . . but I can only find five so it still won't "assemble" and my baby is crying and I don't want my wife to think I can't handle the situation but maybe I shouldn't have just had those two rum and cokes? . . . Is this normal?

The internet provides dads with a sympathetic global audience ready to provide assurance, share their own stories and offer advice. This can be of great comfort as it's good to know that you're not the only guy who missed the memo about how to be a dad.

Shopping for Baby Gear
Once you find out you're going to be a dad, there comes a moment where you look around your place and think, *Oh crap, we're going to need a whole lot of gear* (see Chapter Four).

Once, you were limited to what was available to you on the shelves of any Baby Depot within reasonable driving range of your house on a Sunday afternoon. Buying second-hand stuff through weekly classifieds was also fairly arduous. ("Sorry, you live in Blackdog Springs? Where is that exactly?") The net has made shopping for baby stuff a much less laborious task. It's super easy to compare products and prices, get user reviews, find a bargain or buy second-hand, all from the comfort of your phone or computer, and all delivered to your door. Online grocery shopping can also come as a welcome revelation to the sleep-deprived, time-poor parent.

Disadvantages
Over-Sharing
There is an excitement around pregnancy, childbirth and becoming a parent. Your friends and family will want to know about it, and you will proudly want to tell them. The fact of the matter is, however, that while to you the birth of your child is the biggest thing since the invention of aerosol cheese, to most of your friends, "friends," and family, your parenting adventure is but a thread in life's rich tapestry, taking a back seat in their own equally busy lives.

Social media allows for ease and instantaneous updates, but the savvy new parent needs to be wary not to over-share all the mundane minutiae of one's daily journey. ("Hey, gang, Day 196 and Becky passed her Glucose Challenge Test. Yay! BP is good and cervical plug holding well. We've picked fifty names for the baby. Click _here_ to vote on surveymonkey for your fave!") Because (I mean this nicely) nobody cares.

Cautious restraint is advised. Pregnancy announcement = fine. A few updates along the way (including no more than one ultrasound shot) = fine. Announcement and photos post delivery = absolutely. "Skylar's poop got all the way up to her neck this morning!" = not fine.

If you feel the compulsive need to let everyone know everything (I'm not judging. This would have been me, for sure), at least set up your own blog or lifecast site so friends can opt in rather than be entrapped by your hijacking of their everyday social media.

Information Overload

The internet gives you access to a whole world of information. The sheer volume of it, however, can leave you bamboozled, befuddled and confused.

Type in "Should I circumcise my son?" and you have around 400,000 websites from which to inform your answer. Imagine standing in the middle of a stadium four times the size of Wrigley Field and asking the same question, and having 400,000 voices all yelling at you at the same time. Having so many responses is ironically like having no responses at all.

This is what I refer to as "the spaghetti sauce phenomenon." When I learned to make spaghetti sauce, it was: throw in some meat and tomatoes, onion, garlic, basil, oregano and maybe experiment with celery, carrot, bay leaves, wine and even chili. You can't really go wrong. But, if you look up spaghetti-sauce recipes online, you have around ten million choices to confuse you. Sure, there's something to be said about variety and different ways of doing things, but ten million websites can tend to complicate something that really isn't that complicated in the first place – and be a massive time waster.

I've seen a "how to bathe your baby" website that had a ridiculously detailed, step-by-step guide to baby bathing, complete with diagrams, little animations, links to clips, and complicated instructions. I imagine somewhere some poor guy with his iPad leaning up against the sink trying to follow this through to the letter. Problem is, when there is too much information like this, you can lose faith in your own common sense and judgement and develop a learned helplessness.

The other question that needs to be asked is: do you really need to know *everything*? Sure, it's good to be informed and have some idea of what's going on. But can too much information be a bad thing? Are there some times where ignorance might be bliss?

I have some friends for whom watching YouTube clips of women giving birth didn't really prepare them for the experience as much as cause them anxiety. There used to be almost a wide-eyed wonder for the first-time dad seeing his child come into the world. Has the internet removed some of the mystery and awe around this?

The Level Playing Field

The Pacific Northwest tree octopus is native to the forests around Washington State. After spending its early years in rivers and lakes, it emerges to spend its adult life in the trees. You can read about it online. There are photographs, migratory charts, life-cycle diagrams, expert opinions, mating rituals, appeals to help save it in its endangered state, FAQs, links to related sites . . .

Savvy readers will perhaps raise their eyebrows at the beguiling thought of a tree octopus, and their cynicism would be well founded, as the tree octopus is, of course, a hoax. The now famous Tree Octopus website was created in the late '90s and is frequently used in information-literacy classes to illustrate the power of the internet; namely, that people believe stuff simply because it is published online. It's as if when people sit down in front of a screen, they switch off their discernment meter. There's a webpage, and it looks official and sounds authoritative, so it must be true . . . because it's on the internet.

Here's the problem for the soon-to-be or new parent looking online for information. Let's say you are wondering about circumcising your son. You go online and stumble upon the Circumcision Alliance website. It looks quite official and has a fancy name. It has a logo, links to articles, graphics, statistics, and heartfelt and persuasive arguments for why boys should be routinely circumcised. With the next click, you find yourself in the RACP website. It looks equally official and has a fancy name. It has a logo, links to articles, graphics, statistics, and heartfelt and persuasive arguments for why boys should *not* be routinely circumcised. Herein lies the dilemma. One says potato; the other says p'tah-to. What are you to do? Who do you allow to inform your thoughts?

The internet allows anybody to publish whatever they want (which is simultaneously its great strength and weakness) but this also means that, regardless of background, experience or qualifications, everyone's an expert.

If you were to dig a bit deeper, you would discover that the RACP is the Royal Australasian College of Physicians, an almost hundred-year-old professional body representing about 15,000 pediatricians and physicians across the Tasman, involved in medical education, research, training and advocacy. The equally impressive-sounding Circumcision Alliance turns out to be a guy called Bob who has a bad haircut and a Masters degree purchased off the net. (Just to be clear, the Circumcision Alliance does not exist at the time of writing. I made it up. But if at some point in the future it comes to be, then good luck to it. And to Bob.)

Anyone can create their own website or blog, and even make it look pretty authoritative. But it takes even less effort (the ability to type) to hold court in a parenting forum, which is where you really need to be on your guard. Because in among all the reasonable, measured, helpful advice, you will also get contributions from whackos and dimwits. For example, in an online forum, MummaBop writes the following:

I've held Seana in cars a couple of times without a seatbelt. I always make sure I have a really strong grip, just in case there's an accident. It's not ideal, but I don't have a car and sometimes I just have to do what I have to do.

The seat belt isn't long enough to go around us both, but I'm holding on to her tight. Crushing her isn't an issue. Letting go would be. And I make sure I have a good grip of her AT ALL TIMES . . . so I wouldn't have to react . . . I'm already ready. ATM it's not worth buying a car seat because Seana will outgrow it very quickly.

And DON'T JUDGE ME for it. I'm not an idiot. I KNOW if we were to have an accident there is NO WAY I would let her go.

My response?

MummaBop, thank you for your invitation not to judge you nor find you an idiot. Your request is denied on both counts. Perhaps you would like to go online and read about the hundreds of babies who have died because they weren't strapped in, and whose parents – I'm sure – were just as well meaning as you.

I do not apologize for the above paragraph nor do I wish to make cheap points out of human tragedy. But know this: just because people can type does not give them the right to influence your behavior. The internet gives voice to idiots. It is your job to stay away from them.

Universalizing

The internet is a good and worthy place for new parents to seek out answers to a question or concern they are experiencing. For example, Flynn's wife, Tian, is two weeks overdue so they look online for "natural methods" to promote the onset of labor. They immediately enter a forum where NewMom128 has typed this: "I was two weeks overdue, and a friend suggested I eat pineapple. I ate pineapple and Jonah was born not long after."

A reply from AmazingBu follows: "I ate pineapple for both my births and within minutes I started feeling contractions, so despite what people say, eating pineapple does work!"

A flurry of pineapple-loving comments follows from a variety of moms, all proclaiming the inductive properties of *Ananas comosus*. Faced with this tsunami of support, Flynn and Tian might be forgiven for thinking that pineapple induces labor. The only problem is, it doesn't. (To be fair, fresh pineapple does contain an enzyme – bromelain – which is said to ripen the cervix, but you'd need to eat a truckload of fresh pineapple to possibly have any effect, and by that stage a late labor would be the least of the pregnant woman's concerns.)

Beware of the type of post that suggests "This was my experience so it must be true for everyone." Also, don't be swayed just because nine or ten or fifty other forum responses agree. Just because a handful of people around the world vehemently claim that urinating in a cup of Drano will predict the sex of your child, it does not make it so.

For everyone who posts a tip online, there are ninety-nine for whom the very same thing did not work or who had a totally opposite experience ("I would never go to a public hospital again!" v. "Our public hospital was amazing!"/"Morphine does nothing to ease the pain" v. "Thank you, God, for morphine, which got me through my delivery"/"Jake didn't cry once for any of his vaccinations and now I feel safe knowing he's protected" v. "Our son got vaccinated and almost died" and so on).

While reading about other people's experiences can be informative and even reassuring, bear in mind that just because something did or did not happen to someone else does not necessarily mean it will or will not happen to you.

What to Do?

So here's the rub: the internet is a wonderfully fantastic source of information about pregnancy, childbirth and parenting, but it is imperative that you brace yourself in advance for the flood of qualified and unqualified opinions that will come surging your way. Here are a few things to look out for when perusing a blog, website or forum about dadhood stuff:

- *Who is the author?* I tend to have healthy caution around anything I read online when the author is not identified. Just because someone blogs as "babyguru" does not make them a "baby guru."
- *Other details.* Some websites appear to be an "organization" of some sort, but they seem only to exist in the digital world. Look for other details, such as a postal address and phone number or detailed personnel or organizational information in the "Who are we?" or "Mission statement"-type sections.
- *Quality.* You can usually get a vibe from a website just by looking at its layout, colors, fonts, and so on. Does it look legit or amateurish? If there are typos of grammar or spelling, misuse of apostrophes, headache-inducing color

schemes or massive overuse of exclamation marks or capital letters to make a point, I TEND TO MOVE ON!!!!!!!!!!!

- *Referencing.* When people make sweeping claims, look for a reliably quoted source. For example, I read the following on a "HealthyMomLove" type blog: "Vaccinated children are more chronically ill than unvaccinated children. They have thirty percent higher levels of ADHD, asthma, fainting, allergies, autism, gross motor problems and ear infections." Really, HealthyMomLove? Is there a peer-reviewed, statistically supported and published study from a reputable journal or college that claims this, or is it just your own fanciful conjecture?
- *Authority.* One of the great advantages of Web 2.0 is the "power to the people" concept, that everyone can contribute and share their experiences online. We are no longer excluded from the secretive knowledge of the official or medical world. Parents are now more informed and able to ask questions about their pregnancy and birth. However, while not wanting to go back to blindly accepting what a doctor says (after all, the medical community did once endorse smoking and thalidomide), let's not throw out the baby with the bathwater. I tend to be fairly conservative by nature and I will typically listen more closely to a highly experienced professional who has dedicated most of their life to training, reading, attending conferences and working in their chosen field than to some anonymous blogger with a bee in their bonnet.

So use the internet, but use it well. Dads who use the internet well are sixty times more likely to be good dads. I read that somewhere. Online. So it must be true.

4

Buying Stuff

"The moment you start to think that your baby
needs an Aston Martin, leather-lined, alloy-wheeled
stroller is exactly the time for you to take a long,
hard look at yourself and realize that your baby
doesn't care about brands . . ."

Equipment

Us guys tend to be familiar and okay with accumulating equipment. Whether you're a musician, skier, athlete, chef, home handyman or amateur mechanic, you've probably gathered a stockpile of specialist tools somewhere in your immediate vicinity in the form of various gizmos, bits of gear and do-diddly-whatsits that allow you to do what you like to do with ease, comfort and pleasure.

Being a new parent also requires specialist "baby gear."

Like I did, you probably have some intuitive sense that you'll need some sort of seat thing in the car, a highchair maybe, a crib of sorts . . . But how does this play out? What equipment do you actually need to navigate the next few years of your life as a dad?

First things first: be warned! A quick stroll through your local baby-equipment store or baby expo or online warehouse will leave your head spinning at the almost infinite number of baby-related products, gizmos and accessories available on the market. (Bet you didn't even know there was such a thing as "Nipple Butter," huh?) Don't be bamboozled by all the stuff you see. There is a lot of junk on the market, and you don't actually need all the bits 'n' pieces, so be wary. (A friend of mine suggests you take your grandmother to the Baby Barn and, if she can't identify it, don't buy it. I sort of applaud this in an old-school way, but applying the same criteria would mean kissing goodbye to my Blu-ray player.)

Manufacturers are experts at playing on your naivety and inexperience as a parent, to scare you into thinking that, if you don't have a diaper alarm that plays a melody every time your baby releases a big one, you're negligent. They also play the celebrity-endorsement card, and if you're not on your game, it will suddenly make sense for you to buy this really expensive bassinet because, hey, it's the same one used by [insert here: royal couple, reality TV star, famous actor, rock star, etc.]. So, it must be good, right?

Remember that when Adam and Eve had kids they didn't have all the gadgets and gizmos that we have to have now, and they seem to have survived all right. Even today, millions of families around the world outside the consumerist West raise their children without filling their homes with expensive, color-coordinated baby guff. (How did kids ever survive before baby-crawler knee pads came along?)

When you find yourself picking something up in a baby store and that voice in your head says, *Yeah, this would be good to have,* a good litmus test is to ask whether there are simpler alternatives. Do you really need a hermetically sealed vacuum chamber for diaper disposal, when a plastic bag will do? Do you really need a weeblock to protect yourself from your infant son's urine stream when changing his diaper when you could just use your hand, or a bit of cloth, or, if you really have to, make your own weeblock using say, um, a plastic cup?

Another litmus test is to ask, *Who am I really buying this for?* The moment you start to think that your baby needs an Aston Martin, leather-lined, alloy-wheeled stroller is exactly the time for you to take a long, hard look at yourself and realize that your baby doesn't care about brands, as long as the thing feels comfortable and is safe.

Having said that, of course, we live where we live and so there will naturally be a degree to which we will want or "need" what are considered the "basics" in our culture. But at least go into it with your eyes open. Pause and think. Be selective and wise in your stockpiling. Before you go off on a mortgage-busting spree, sit down with your wife and work out what you need and what you can afford.

If you're planning on having a few children, it's probably more economical to buy, either new or second-hand. But if you don't want to outlay the cash up front, some items can be rented. Remember, too, that some things might be given to you as presents. Or maybe you have friends who are just finishing their own baby saga and are willing and ready to off-load some of their gear onto you.

In this era of sustainability and recycling, the classifieds and internet provide access to a wealth of second-hand goods.

When buying second-hand or online, always ensure that it conforms to current safety standards. Be particularly vigilant for equipment that doesn't cut the mustard; you don't want your baby having anything to do with cheap, shonky or dangerous products. The Consumer Product Safety Commission website has copious amounts of detailed and valuable information (i.e., the available-online "Baby Seat Car Pouch" looks legit on a website but doesn't come close to current standards and you'd be better off tying your baby to the back seat with a pair of old athletic socks).

Another thing. And this is an important one.

Avoid the trap of buying stuff simply because it suits your decor or because you're trying to live up to some sort of baby-magazine, designer-photo-spread ideal. I know a couple who bought one of those old-style English nanny prams because they thought they would look cute going for a walk in the park with it. The stroller did look great in a retro kind of way . . . but it didn't fold up well, so they couldn't put it in their car, and it didn't store easily. It was also next to impossible to clean. And it had terrible suspension and the baby didn't appear comfortable in it. But, hey, at least they *looked* good.

So, whatever you buy, make sure:

- it is strong and sturdy and made out of robust materials
- it is storable and will fit into your home somewhere
- your baby can't swallow it
- that after you buy it you still have enough money for food for the rest of the week
- it is washable – preferably capable of withstanding a hose-down in the backyard.

Some products come certified with an International Radiation Symbol sticker. This means it has survived a nuclear explosion and, as such, has a good chance of making it through six months of use with a baby.

If you're still stuck in figuring out what to buy and what not to buy, get your hands on a copy of the latest edition of *The Choice Guide to Baby Products* or visit the Consumer Product Safety Commission website.

Below is a collection of some other ramblings from my own experiences with baby equipment that you might find helpful.

Baby Zone

Your baby needs a place to live.

Current advice is that your baby sleeps at night in a crib in your room for the first six to twelve months. Counterintuitively, it is reported that parents sleep better because they can check on the baby by just rolling over, rather than getting up and padding down the corridor and waking up and then, oh, well, while I'm up, I'll turn on the lights and check my emails and update my status ("3 am and little Jake is snug as a bug . . ."). Parents reportedly like the security of knowing that the baby is nearby and feel that it provides more comfort and closeness for their baby, rather than it being all alone in some dark, quiet room somewhere. I know some people for whom this works well, and others who did it for a few weeks but found it exhausting because they woke up every time the baby moved (or, ironically, *didn't* move), and they became paranoid about making noise themselves. And another couple for whom it was a disaster, so the husband went and slept in a separate room.

I also know one couple who decided to have their baby not only in their own room but in their bed with them. This is not exactly my cup of kopi luwak, and no authority recommends this (i.e., don't do it) because of the risk of the baby getting lost in the sheets and blankets, the risk of it falling out or sliding down and getting trapped between a wall and the bed, and the risk of a heavy sleeper (or parent who has had a few drinks) rolling on them.

Personally, I like my own space and think it is a good idea for a baby to have its own space too. There should be some place where you won't be disturbed by it too much – say, for example, Brazil.

Our babies were born and raised in an era where it was okay to have them elsewhere in the house. (Then again, this was also the same era when both the public caning of children in schools and smoking in restaurants were okay.) We were fortunate in that we had a spare bedroom next to ours that we could convert into a nursery. If you are going to make a similar conversion, whatever you do, don't look at the pictures of nurseries in baby magazines, especially if it's a home feature about a Hollywood starlet or pop singer or the word "Supermom" is used anywhere in the by-line. These have been designed by architects, outfitted by interior decorators and photographed by professionals in the homes of millionaires. Using actors and models.

The nurseries of us mere mortals in the real world are small, cramped, messy and smell of ammonia.

When Georgia came along, we had run out of rooms to convert into another nursery and it wasn't practical to put her in with Rachael. So we converted part of the hallway into a bedroom. (When she got older, she became roommates with Rachael while Matilda took over the hallway spot.) And, by the way, all our kids turned out okay.

No matter where your baby goes, there are a few bits and pieces that will make life a lot easier: a fan or heater help to control the extremes of temperature, and a comfortable chair with a rug and footstool are nice for night-time feeds if feeding in bed is impractical.

Sleeping Zone

New babies need a place to sleep. Normal-sized beds are too big. They should go into a bassinet, cradle or cot, something nice and cozy.

Be careful not to get sucked into baby-magazine fantasy advertising. A Colonial-style cedar crib with decorative carvings and lace coverings may look beautiful, but it will cost you a fortune. And if you think the baby gives a stuff about the aesthetics of its crib, think again.

Because of the risk of SIDS, the baby's sleeping space should be free of bits 'n' pieces, such as loose bedclothes, quilts, blankets, pillows, stuffed toys, bumpers, water bottles and electric blankets.

Some cradles rock. These can be useful in swaying babies off to sleep, but make sure they don't swing like the pirate-ship ride at an amusement park. Babies don't like being upside down. It is recommended that a cradle does not swing more than ten degrees from its static position (i.e., a swing you could do with a gentle push with one finger).

As your baby gets bigger, a crib will be more suitable for its nocturnal wrigglings. The crib must have tall sides so your baby won't fall or climb out of it. It must have a mattress that can withstand multiple rinsings in toxic bodily fluids. And, if it has wheels, they should be lockable.

Don't be tempted to paint the crib. Your baby will soon grow razor-like teeth, and it will spend a great deal of time gnawing away at the bars. And paint is *not* one of the five major food groups.

Another necessity is one of those wind-up musical gizmos designed for soothing babies off to sleep. Unfortunately, the only tune available on the market is Brahms' *Lullaby.* You know the one. It goes, "Da-da-daa, da-da-daa, da-da daa-daa-da-daa-daa." Brahms was a sadist, and you will come to hate this tune. Oh yes. You will.

Clothing

Babies are tiny and they need their own special, tiny clothes: onesies, booties, beanies, coveralls/jumpsuits, matinee jackets, tees and nighties, depending on the weather. Most babies start off in a size 000, which isn't too much bigger than something you would dangle off your key ring.

As they get older, you will need to expand and upgrade their wardrobe at a breathtaking rate. Make sure you purchase items for practical reasons, as opposed to making a fashion statement. Having said that, don't run off to the shops straight

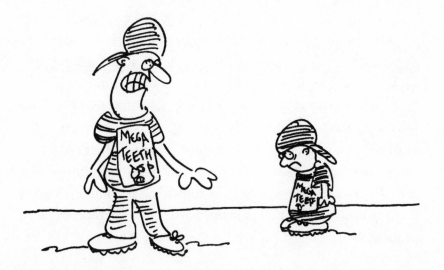

away. Clothes are a standard newborn present from your friends and family. When Rachael was born, we used a shovel to move all the clothes she got as presents. In fact, she got so many that Georgia and Matilda were set for years of hand-me-downs.

There is one disadvantage to hand-me-downs. Now, when I flip through our family photos, I can't tell which of my kids is which because they're all dressed the same.

Changing Zone

When changing or dressing babies, you will need a panoply of items, including diapers, snappies (if using cloth), undies, lotions, creams, wipes, plastic bags, liners, tissues, a gasmask, welding gloves and an industrial furnace to destroy any contaminants. It's best to establish a spot somewhere where all this paraphernalia can be centralized and contained.

You can always use the floor as a change space, but this means getting up and down like a jack-in-the-box all day. Friends of mine just put a towel out on their bed or couch. If you have the space, you could invest in a freestanding changing table that has shelves for all the bits and pieces and a comfortable mat on top for the baby. If you buy one, make sure it is sturdy.

The main problem with changing tables is that they are designed for hobbits. If you stand over six foot like me, that slight and sustained awkward stoop every few hours will give your physical therapist enough regular income to keep their kids in private school for years to come. An alternative that worked very well for us was a simple foam mat that we sat on top of the baby's chest of drawers. This was high enough for me (thanks to a couple of bricks under the legs) and it meant that we didn't need to clutter up the room with another piece of furniture.

A word of warning, though: newborns are pretty docile in that they haven't yet figured out how to wriggle, twist and claw their way away from you while you're trying to change or dress them. But, as they get older, they develop a lemming-like ability to throw themselves off changing tables. Never leave a baby unattended on a changing table – not even for a second. Get all the stuff ready *before* you put the baby on the table. If you have to turn away to get something, keep one hand firmly planted on the baby at all times.

Again, in case you have started skim-reading . . . Never leave a baby unattended on a changing table – not even for a second. Get all the stuff ready *before* you put the baby on the table. If you have to turn away to get something, keep one hand firmly planted on the baby at all times.

Baby Monitor

If the nursery is a distance from your bedroom or main living area, you can get a baby monitor so that, when you hear the baby cry, you can switch it off. But if you live in an apartment or house like other mere mortals, just use your ears.

And unless you live in some sort of resort complex, mansion or private high-rise, I am especially not a fan of video monitoring systems – another over-the-top, un-necessity of the baby-marketing era. I've seen one advertised as sporting five cameras, six-meter night vision, full HD sound, remote lullaby control and zoom capability broadcasting to four split screens on your tablet or TV. It's even wi-fi based, so you can "check on baby when you're out and about," with a graphic of mom and dad at a restaurant, laughing and drinking wine while looking at their baby from four angles on a smartphone. Correct me if I'm wrong, but if there's a babysitter at home, these parents need to "let go" and stop with the Big Brother surveillance. And if there's *not* a babysitter at home, they need to go home. Either way, this is uncool.

To be fair, though, some people swear by these things. Friends of mine received a video monitor as a gift. They were at first disdainful, but now swear by it, their main argument being that they can actually check on their baby without going into the room, which in itself can lead to the baby waking up or getting excited at your arrival.

Lighting

In the first weeks, you will probably check on your baby quite a lot during the night. This is of course assuming that you can *see* the baby. To a sleeping baby, an ordinary ceiling light is like a 747 landing on its face, and it will not be happy.

A simple, inexpensive night-light (or a video monitoring system, as above) will solve the problem. These are very small, soft lights that are so low in intensity they don't even register on your electricity meter. They allow midnight checkings without midnight awakenings and will save your toes from midnight collisions.

Decorations

It's funny how the decor of your home changes once you have a child. Our place started out with stylemeister black-and-white photographs and arty prints. Then, somewhere along the way, they got replaced by illustrative alphabet posters. (A is for Aardvark and X is for Xylophone, in case you were wondering.)

It's nice to decorate your baby's space so that it is colorful and stimulating. There are countless posters and friezes out there, showcasing a variety of cute animals, numbers, letters and nursery-rhyme characters.

I Blu-tacked a *Terminator* poster in the "nursery" while Meredith was in the hospital. When she got home with our newborn, she was not happy.

Don't do this.

That was not a night I care to remember.

Stuffed Toys

Sometimes in the middle of the night I am besieged by important-at-the-time-but-not-so-much-the-next-morning questions, such as:

- Who *really* shot JFK? (Seriously, once you've stood at that window in the Book Depository, you know it wasn't Oswald.)
- Why do hot dogs make good sense as a foodstuff at 1 am?
- What are the Colonel's eleven herbs and spices?
- When Walt Disney comes back from being cryonically frozen, would he like *Star Wars*?

And this: why are there so many stuffed toys in our house?

We have at various points had, no kidding, hundreds of them: stuffed bunnies, stuffed bears, stuffed cats, stuffed ducks, stuffed cows, stuffed donkeys, stuffed monkeys, stuffed penguins, stuffed pigs, stuffed dogs, stuffed ABC Kids and Disney movie characters, and every kind of stuffed marsupial imaginable. From the giant stuffed gorilla (#cryingkids) through to the mini stuffed alien that came with a drive-thru hamburger meal, we've had them all.

Worse still, most of them squeak or have jingly bells or a "Press My Chest" button, causing them to say something cute. And, trust me, if you want to know the real meaning of fear, it's waking at 2:30 am to a stuffed-toy robotic voice coming down the hallway in the quiet darkness declaring, "I'm gon-na give you a haircut."

Here's the thing. We didn't buy any stuffed toys. They were all gifts. And I'm pretty sure we only started with about twenty. So ... where did they all come from? Clearly ... they're breeding. Every night, there's a stuffed-toy party in the cupboard and they are producing their own stuffed-toy spawn and are planning the conquest of our house.

Don't buy stuffed toys. They will end up in your house anyway.

Also, keep stuffed toys out of the baby's crib or cot. It's fine to have them on a bookshelf or windowsill, but, despite how awesome they look in photographs, all the advice from SIDS prevention bodies is to keep them well away from sleeping spaces. Aside from restricting airflow, they are just scary as hell to a baby.

Hygiene
Bath
Babies need to be cleaned. However, they're not very good at doing it themselves.

Your baby can either hop in the bath with you or, since they're so small, you can bathe them in a sink or the laundry tub. We didn't have a suitable sink, and our first home didn't have a bath, so we bought a small, plastic bath. These are readily available, inexpensive and can be put on a sturdy and safe kitchen or bathroom counter. To accompany the bath, you will also end up buying an assortment of washcloths, towels and squeaky toys, all plastered with cute, ducky motifs.

Assorted Bits and Pieces

There are many little bits and pieces you will need to have with you when bathing or changing your baby. I'm not sure what they're all for, but since everyone else seems to have them in their baby's nurseries, you don't want to look negligent.

You need baby oil, olive oil, bath oil, engine oil, baby lotion, baby powder, a lambskin rug, an old stocking stuffed with oatmeal (don't ask), washcloths, baby shampoo, zinc cream, a soft brush, cotton balls, cotton swabs, tissues, methylated spirits, soft towels, a comb and several jars of unidentifiable, lumpy grey stuff.

Feeding

Bottles and Things

To feed a baby, you need:

- two milk-swollen breasts, or
- a can or jar of milk formula with a bottle kit.

Later, you'll need:

- a pantry full of powdered cereals, fruit gels, yogurts and purées
- a collection of cute baby placemats, tablecloths, crockery and cutlery
- a highchair (see below).

Here's something I didn't know before we had children: breast-milk can be bottled too. This raises the question: how do you get it into the bottle in the first place? You use a breast pump, of course. When I heard the words "breast pump" for the first time, I had visions of Meredith entangled in the irrigation pump on my Uncle George's farm – a huge, greasy, diesel beast that smokes and coughs noisily in the corner of his shed.

Fortunately, breast pumps aren't like this. They are small and dainty. You can get manual ones, which are like wide-mouthed syringes, or electric ones with a little motor. Once some milk has been "expressed," it can be stored and labelled in plastic bags or ice-cube trays and frozen for later use. Your wife can build up a supply over a period of time. This is very useful for the babysitter if you and your wife go out. Of course, as with using formula, you need to buy an assortment of bottles, nipples and a sterilizing kit. When the baby gets older, the bottles can be used for water or juice.

Breastfeeding is recommended as the baby's sole source of food for the first six months, to be continued as per mother and baby preference with other foods for up to two years. Of course, you can go beyond that, as long as you know that your friends will get weirded out if your wife "boobs up" for your child between innings of their Little League game.

Bouncer

As our babies grew, we found a bouncer was a great way to get them off the floor and sitting semi-upright so they could have a look at what was going on in the world around them, while providing us with a few precious moments of having two hands to do stuff, such as chop vegetables. Please note my use of the word "floor" in the sentence above. Bouncers are only for use on the floor and should never, ever be put on a countertop or table. As the name suggests, they are just too likely to bounce off.

Be careful, though, not to inadvertently tread on the back of the bouncer and then suddenly release it in surprise, unless you want to give your baby a quick lesson in the physics of medieval siege warfare.

Highchair

About the time babies sit up by themselves, they can also start on more "solid" foods. But don't misconstrue this milestone as meaning you can just pop them up at your table, because they'll disappear through the cracks in your dining-room furniture.

A highchair is a good investment. The baby can join you for dinner at the table so all your dinner guests have a good view when it dumps a plate of spaghetti on its head.

Make sure the highchair is cleanable (suggest purchase of high-pressure water cleaner), strong (it won't collapse), secure (it has a harness so your baby can't make like Houdini from it) and has no folding or closing mechanisms that could trap fingers or toes.

Transport and Mobility

Babies can't walk.

They don't even crawl for six or seven months, or even longer.

Even once they learn to crawl, they are still pretty slow. Something as simple as going to the corner shop will take you hours – to say nothing of the damage done to the baby's knees. So modern baby-gear designers have come to the rescue by inventing many accessories for baby transport.

Car Travel

Kids must be restrained in cars. Strapping them into adult seatbelts doesn't work (they just keel over) and invites police fines and obvious disaster in the event of an accident. I was horrified to see a Molly Ringwald film once (I could just finish that part of the sentence there . . .) in which she holds a newborn baby in her lap in the front seat of a car. I thought this an unrealistic twist of fiction but, unbelievably, some parents do this. I know this because they post their confessionals online. ("It wasn't like a road trip or anything . . . it was just to the mall. LOL!" #shouldnthavehadchildren.)

If you are traveling at thirty-five miles an hour with your baby unrestrained and you crash, you will not be able to hold it. It would be the same as dropping your baby from a second-story window onto concrete. And putting it in your seatbelt with you is worse. The physics of your body rapidly decelerating from thirty-five miles an hour would provide a crushing several tons of force on your baby. (Think: elephant treading on baby.)

By law, you must have specialized baby/child seating for around the first seven to eight years. Child passenger safety laws vary somewhat from state to state, but in general, kids must ride in the backseat whenever possible. Look online to find the exact rules—the guidelines that follow may be different in your area.

For the first twelve months (or until it is twenty pounds), your baby must have a rear-facing car seat. The inner chamber of some car seats detaches to make a convenient baby carrier – convenient for short periods of time, anyway. If you don't want to buy a car seat, rent one. These used to be pretty simple plastic shells with a ridiculously fat Velcro strap. Now, they are elaborate, padded survival chambers with body harnesses – the kind of escape pod that Jor-El strapped his infant son Kal-El into for his journey from Krypton to Earth.

When your baby gets a bit older, it will graduate to the dizzy heights of a child safety seat (a molded plastic seat complete with racing harness, which itself is strapped to the car seat) and then finally (from four years) a booster seat, which is a cloth-covered, molded, foam seat that uses only the car's seatbelt as a restraint. If you are buying a second-hand car seat, check that it hasn't been involved in an accident or is otherwise damaged. Check for frayed straps, casing cracks and signs of vomit or other unsightly bodily fluid stains on the fabric.

Massively variable statistics from a range of organizations suggest that anywhere between twenty and seventy percent of baby/child restraints are not fitted correctly, which means they won't do their job effectively in an accident. There are heaps of accredited fitting stations that will fit them for you – either for free or a small charge. Look them up online.

If you drive an old-model vehicle, check that it has a restraining-bolt hole on which to attach the rear strap. You need this to secure both car seats and seats. When Rachael was born, we were driving an ancient van that didn't have a bolt hole, so we had to have a bar fitted across the back.

Don't wait until the day your baby is due to leave the hospital to awkwardly discover that your car seat isn't properly fitted into your car. Go and sort it out now. Well? Go on, then.

By the way, while we're talking about cars ... you're gonna need a bigger one. No matter what you drive now, it's not big enough to carry around all the crap you'll need over the coming years.

Diaper Bag

Whenever you go out with a baby, you need to take a survival kit called a diaper bag with you. We had one that we called The Tardis, because it was bigger on the inside than it appeared on the outside, and it held more crap than the laws of physics dictated it should.

Our Tardis bag had everything a baby would need: sunscreen, diapers, plastic pants, snappies, hats, pacifiers, bottles, tissues, cotton swabs, those wet-wipe things, spare clothing, books, soft toys, jars of slushy food, spoons, bibs, plastic bags, lambskin rug, orienteering compass, capsicum spray, Armalite MH-12 Maghook and a radio distress beacon.

Stroller

Babies may be small, but they get heavy after a while. You can't simply carry them all the time. Being on wheels, a stroller allows you to transport your baby around without having to bear too much weight yourself.

With our climate, it is important to find a stroller that will provide shade for the baby. Some strollers have extendable hoods or umbrella attachments, but you should at the very least be able to jerry-rig a towel on it to provide cover.

The stroller we bought cost us more than my first car. It also had more features: eight rotating wheels, a reclining seat, four-way wheel-locks (a very important safety feature), independent steering, full reversibility, luggage compartment, shade hood, rain hood, compression shocks, adjustable handles, seatbelt harnesses, running-boards and *Ben Hur* chariot wheels that could easily shred the ankles of anyone stupid enough to get in our way. It could do almost twenty miles an hour with a tailwind without getting speed-wobbles, it was light to push, comfortable for the baby, easy to clean, and we could fold it up without watching an instructional video.

The newer style of jogger strollers have become very popular in recent years. You have no doubt seen these, as they whiz past you on the sidewalk in front of some chiselled parent in lycra. These three-wheel joggers are designed for more robust travel, as evidenced by the fact that they look like robotic, all-terrain vehicles from Mars expeditions. They have large, pneumatic tires, sprung suspension, padded passenger modules, alloy tubing, racing harnesses, coffee-cup and smartphone holders at the back, rain hoods designed to withstand cyclones, and GPS satellite capability. They are made out of tough, camping-style material and have bold and adventurously inspiring names such as Terrain, Explorer, Pioneer and Commander. Such vehicles are great if you want to take your baby for a walk along, say, the Appalachian Trail.

You will use your stroller a lot. Get a good one.

Baby Carrier

There are some places where a stroller is impractical, such as on Denali. Also, if you take your baby to the supermarket, you will need one hand to get things off the shelves, one hand to push the cart and one hand to carry the baby or push a stroller. That makes three hands, which is a problem for most people.

You can take the baby in its car seat and place it in the shopping cart, although, aside from being pretty unstable, this will leave you only enough room in your cart to buy two tins of soup and a stick of celery. This is where baby carriers and slings come in quite handy. A baby carrier, which you wear on your chest, is useful for little babies, while the backpack is more suitable for bigger ones.

At first, I thought we could just stuff our baby inside the backpack I'd taken around Europe. After all, it was very spacious, had a strong frame and many colorful cloth badges

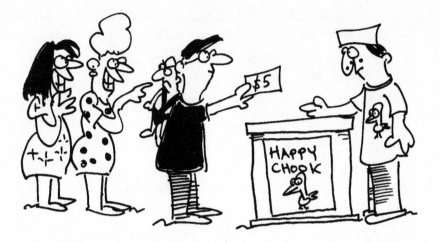

from places of interest that I had visited. However, Rachael didn't like it very much, and people in the street looked at me like I was some kind of weirdo. So we bought a carrier with good padding and straps. Your baby faces you so it's like you are cuddling and you can have a chat as you stroll along. These are great for an outing to the zoo, or a walk to the shops, pool or park. They also work well in the screamy hours when you are trying to get your baby off to sleep. The rocking motion works for them, and getting out of the confines of your home works for you.

As your baby gets bigger, the back carrier is better, where the baby sits up high behind you, allowing it to get a good view of the action and also show what it thinks of you by dribbling on your head and yanking huge handfuls of your hair. Framed seats like this are not recommended for babies under four months.

Some mothers like a more traditional wrap or front-slung sling (try saying *that* after a few chardonnays), like the mothers in *National Geographic*. These are essentially a long, stretchy piece of fabric that you wrap around your body in a complicated way and then tuck the baby inside. They allow for intimate contact with the baby (and breastfeeding on the run) while keeping your two hands free for doing whatever it is your two hands want to be doing – washing, texting, cleaning, vacuuming, cooking or rappeling. But if you have trouble tying anything more complex than a reef knot, then this is not for you. While slings are okay if worn correctly, there are significant dangers if not. I strongly suggest you read the latest information and advice from the Consumer Product Safety Commission. And to be honest, I haven't really seen these take off with the dads.

Baby Walker

Look, I'm not too impressed by these and my advice to you is to steer well clear. They look cute in ads, but walkers give babies a mobility they may not be ready for – like giving a ten-year-old the keys to your car. In a walker, a baby gains the capacity to travel around your house at approximately twenty miles an hour and use their vehicle as a battering ram. A walker also helps the baby to stand upright and reach expensive and forbidden domestic equipment.

I'm from the old school that believes babies will walk when they're good and ready, and that it's a bit pretentious to push them. Babies put in walkers get used to the support they provide and are slower in becoming independent walkers. More importantly, walkers are dangerous. Houses are too full of stairs and inclines and sharp corners and electric cords to accommodate aspiring Formula One drivers.

Baby Door Jumper

These are seats or harnesses that hang suspended under a doorframe, generally with a spring or elastic-type rope, allowing the baby to jump and bounce on the spot. It sort of looks cute, but these are held in universal disregard by baby experts and consumer-safety organizations. Aside from promoting developmental delay (à la walkers), there is too much risk of fingers getting caught or kids falling out of them.

My darkly comedic side can't help but think that it should surely be counter-intuitive to load a baby into a spring-based mechanism with two launching ropes pointed at a doorframe. I have visions of either the baby firing upwards, leaving a head-shaped divot in the architrave, or the doorframe collapsing down with elasticized velocity onto said child. Neither eventuality ends up well, really.

Playpen

As opposed to strollers and backpacks and slings (which are all designed to enhance baby mobility), a playpen is designed to do exactly the opposite; namely, enforce baby *im*mobility.

When babies get a bit older, they like to move around the house searching for things to destroy or chew. It can be difficult to monitor their movements every second, and sometimes a frustrated parent needs just a couple of minutes to go to the toilet or boil an egg or brush their hair or put on a pair of socks or complete a tax return. Which is where a playpen is handy.

If you get a playpen, use your common sense. Look for strength and stability so that it can't collapse or tip over. Watch out for splinters, toxic paint, sharp edges, finger-jamming hinges and head-trapping bars. Even then, don't assume that your baby's relative lack of mobility allows you to leave it unsupervised. Just think of your carpet.

Physical Therapist

Okay, technically a professional practitioner is not an item of baby gear. But now's as good a time as any to tell you the following: being a dad wrecks your back. You're gonna need a good physical therapist.

While this may seem a cheap space-filler, it's not. For the next few years, you will put your spine, lats, pecs, biceps and forearms through all sorts of contortions: rocking a little dead-weight package off to sleep on a cold, dark night, leaning into your car with arms outstretched awkwardly to affix said package into car seat, pulling travel cribs and strollers out of car trunks, hunching over changing tables and baths at crippling angles, walking around the zoo or shopping center with one (or two or more?) heavy little humans hanging somewhere off your body, to say nothing of all the time you will spend on intimate terms with the floor, which is where babies and toddlers tend to live.

It's not a matter of *if*, it's a matter of *when* your back is going to go . . . maybe a nice little C3/C4 spasm, or an L2/L3 sciatic pinch, maybe even a herniated disc?

My advice? Yoga, gym, regular exercise, core-strength conditioning, strong posture and a good physical therapist who can crack your spine like dropping a xylophone.

Don't say I didn't warn you.

The Bill

So where exactly does all this "having a baby" thing leave you financially over the next few years? With a house stacked to the creaking rafters with baby junk (and a new physical therapist!).

Here's a rough breakdown:

Lost income	$200,000
Hospital and medical bill	$5,000
Minivan (second-hand)	$30,000
Extensions to house	$150,000
Childcare	$66,000
Bedroom furniture	$3,000
Preschool	$5,000
Swimming lessons	$3,000
Ballet lessons	$1,500
Ballet shoes	$250
Soccer cleats	$90
All other shoes	$850
Excess water bill	$800
Food thrown onto floor	$1,000
Stroller	$600
Car seat	$400
Booster seat	$150
Diapers	$3,000
Baby bath	$80
Baby bath thermometer	$15
Indestructible cutlery and crockery	$150
Carpet shampoo	$400
Plumber (when diaper goes down the toilet)	$650
Jewelry lost by inquisitive toddler	$3500
Baby video monitoring system	$220
Aspirin	$200
iPotty	$60
Cost of a healthy, happy baby	$Priceless

As you are starting to realize, raising children is not cheap. According to estimates from the U.S. Department of Agriculture, it will cost an estimated $241,080, on average, for a middle-income couple to raise a kid from birth to eighteen (based on expenses for housing, food, transportation, clothes, health care, and education—but not including the cost of college). That number gets much higher if you live in an urban area.

It's pretty easy to look at that dollar figure and be put off. Don't be. Sure, having kids will reduce your disposable income for the next bit of your life, but so what? Kids have always been an expense. Your parents were expensive for *their* parents. You were expensive for *your* parents. Now it's your turn. Besides, apart from a few big-ticket items, remember that the expense is spread out day by day and week by week over many years. It's not like you have to write the check on the day they're born. And anyway, what else are you going to spend your money on? Your train set? Nice clothes? A convertible? A home keg-beer system? That nice guitar? Those skis you've had your eye on? Having kids is a good and worthwhile thing to spend your money on. In fact, flip the other way and realize that, rather than it being a burden, you will actually *want* to spend money on your child and provide for it and give it the best. Think of it as a very, very worthwhile investment in the future.

Before we leave the subject of shopping, here's a final word of advice. Watch out for total strangers who accost you at supermarkets who, upon spotting your pregnant wife, descend en masse to rub their hands all over her swollen frontage as if she were public property.

"Having a baby?" they coo. "Oooh, lover-ly, lover-ly. My, he's a big one. Is he going to kick? Are you going to kick, little baby? Goodness me, what a big kick!" And then they lean in and whisper conspiratorially, "I had three littl'uns myself, dear . . . terrible hemorrhoids, and with my third! Well! A seventy-two-hour labor, lost a third of my body weight in blood, and . . . oh, can you believe the price of bananas at the moment?" And, just like that, they're gone.

I'm glad this behavior is reserved for pregnant women. I would not like a complete stranger in the supermarket grabbing a handful of my squiddly-dangles and saying "Oooh, lover-ly, lover-ly."

5

Time to Get Ready

"An eerie silence fell over the room. Strangely out of context, a cricket chirped. We moved on, but none of us were ever the same again."

Study Up

In 1830, Sir Walter Scott wrote to a friend, "All men who have turned out worth anything have had the chief hand in their own education." This applies particularly to fatherhood. My gut feeling is that most guys are like I was in my "pre-dad life"; that is, despite some whimsical notions about wanting to be "a good dad," they don't actually know what this means. They don't have the faintest idea about pregnancy, labor or caring for a baby.

If you want to be a good dad – nay, an *excellent* dad – then you have to be active and involved. You can't simply tag along, watching from the sidelines while you Instagram the best bits of your day. You need to start asking important questions. What happens during pregnancy? What's childbirth like? How do you look after a baby anyway? Did I remember to put the trash out? How can I support my wife? What happens if I faint? And how exactly did my wife get pregnant in the first place?

In short, as Scott said, if you want to be of any worth as a father, start educating yourself. Education – in the form of reading books, chatting with other dads, and engaging with various websites, blogs, communities and whatever other social media exists at the time you read this – will achieve three things.

First, it will help you understand the language used by medical professionals. For example: "Excuse me, sir, a nuchal scan of the episiotomy caused a Caesarean epidural reaction with the zygote and I'm afraid your forceps were cervixed in the panic. As a consequence, our fetal monitor bonded with the ultrasound. Colostrum should do the trick, but if you're still concerned, pop on that cradle cap there and mop the pelvic floor. And, in the name of King and Country, I declare these . . . the Glands of Montgomery!"

Second, it will help you prepare for what's coming your way; for instance, what happens when you go to the hospital and to what extent your life will be different from now on.

Third, it will help to fortify you against the experience of the birth itself.

Tom Hopman was a boy in my Personal Development class at high school. I remember him because, when we watched a film about pregnancy and childbirth, his eyelids fluttered and his body went stiff and he slid off his chair and hit the floor. This drove our class into a rabid frenzy like something out of *Lord of the Flies* – perhaps the reason why I never got to see any of those films in their entirety and why I was therefore an ignoramus about childbirth.

When Meredith was pregnant the first time, I had not seen much in the way of real childbirth before. (And by "not much," I actually mean "nothing.") Sure, I'd seen plenty of *portrayals* of childbirth in Hollywood dramas and comedies (see Appendix I). But these tend to be wildly unrealistic, clichéd and often just plain wrong. Have you seen the real deal? If you have already started at birth class, odds are on that they've shown you some footage of an actual birth already.

The internet, of course, provides a wealth of material in this regard and, as it turns out, YouTube features other things besides skateboarding idiots falling down stairs. For the first time in history, soon-to-be dads have access to thousands of clips of real women giving real birth to real babies, before they encounter it themselves. Personally, I'm not sure *why* women would not only film but then post footage of their labors to the world, but I assume it is for altruistic reasons.

There are a number of other ways you can start learning. The very fact you are reading these words is a sign that you have made a start (even though it is likely this book was given to you by your wife or mother). Well done! However, no single book or blog or website will give you all the answers. My advice is to read – or at least browse through – as many worthy books and magazines and websites as you can. Find some good dad-blogs, where the writer seems measured and real. Practices and beliefs relating to pregnancy, childbirth and parenting can be quite different overseas and they can change over time, so try to stick to the most recent material that is most relevant to you. Also, newsagents have an entire shelf devoted to childbirth and parenting magazines. You can spot them because they have those soft-focus shots of mothers on the cover.

An important step in your education is to familiarize yourself with the place where your wife is going to have the baby.

If you are planning on a home birth, there is a lot of information online about the preparations that need to be made and the long list of gear you should have on hand. (Your midwife will also supply you with this.) If you're planning on a water birth, you might want to test how long it takes to blow up the pool, 'cause if you think you are going to do it with your own lungs once your wife goes into labor, you are kidding yourself, Jack.

Hospitals run tours of the labor and maternity wards, which you can schedule a month or two before the due date. During these tours, a nurse will run through the sequence of events likely to occur from the time you and your wife arrive at the hospital to the time mom and baby are happily recovering in the maternity ward and dad is sleeping soundly on the chair in the corner. You are shown the place to report to, the waiting rooms, the delivery unit and the maternity rooms. You'll see all the high-tech equipment and the low-tech equipment and have an opportunity to ask questions. You also get to find out where the really important things are, such as the restrooms, shop and cafe. It's also worth noting where the parking lot or drop-off bays are in case you're in a hurry.

On our first tour, one young guy pointed at a large, silvery bucket at the base of a bed in the delivery suite. "What's that for?" he queried.

There was a pause.

"Slops," said the midwife, deadpan.

Several men were visibly shaken by this response. An eerie silence fell over the room. Strangely out of context, a cricket chirped. We moved on, but none of us were ever the same again.

Many hospitals offer virtual tours of their maternity centers, so you can visit without leaving the house. Hospitals are also a good source for pamphlets and brochures about various parenting issues and information about support organizations.

Many hospitals and a range of private organizations also offer childbirth-education classes. The most popular types of birth class – Lamaze, Bradley, Alexander, and Mongan – in their own way all work towards similar ends: reducing fear, processing pain, developing skills, encouraging confidence and preparing parents to take in their stride the many directions a birth can take. In Australia, there's even a childbirth-education organization now running childbirth programs for dads in pubs. For me – and my guess is that for many other guys – these classes are an important and primary source of information about the birthing process.

Our classes ran for six consecutive Tuesday nights, although some are done over a couple of Saturdays or as a weekend retreat. For a no-idea guy like me, our classes were great in providing information and reassurance. We learned about pregnancy and labor, listened to talks, watched clips, drew pictures, looked at PowerPoints and stuffed plastic babies through plastic pelvic bones. We did breathing exercises and panted at each other. We took off our shoes and learned about coping with contractions. We rolled around on the floor, screamed, slapped our thighs and swayed back and forth. We practiced back massages and discussed options for pain relief. I learned about being a support person for Meredith.

We asked questions and practiced birthing positions. We leaned into beanbags, squatted down and crawled around on all fours. On the final night, one of the moms from the maternity ward came down and gave us a baby-bathing demonstration – with a real live baby and everything!

There is a certain sense of redundancy in doing some of these activities and exercises, because, as a man, obviously you're not the one having the baby. However, it does help you to get into the mindset of childbirth and also break down any barriers of awkwardness or embarrassment you might be feeling about trying to support a woman who is growling and gnashing her teeth at you.

So get into it! Read books, chat with new dads, search the internet, watch DVDs and go to classes. It's the only way you'll learn.

To Plan or Not to Plan?

In the old days, a pregnant woman had little say in what happened during her labor. She was merely there as a baby incubator, and the labor set-up was arranged for the convenience of the doctor. Supposedly, this is why many women gave birth in the Universal Television Birthing Position (UTBP) – flat on their backs with their feet up in stirrups. It was nice and handy for the doctor. In reality, this is the worst possible childbirth position. Also, the horse tends to get in the way. (I apologize. I couldn't help it.)

Recent years have seen a growing resistance to the UTBP, along with the view that women are just the passive incubators. Women are encouraged to be empowered and knowledgeable about the impending birth, and to participate in the decision-making process. This is a good thing.

But, like most good things, you can go too far.

Some couples work out a birth plan. They do a bit of reading in books and online, discuss the options available in the birth process and then custom-design their own "ideal" birth. The plan might consist of a series of wish-list statements, such as:

- I want to use a beanbag.
- I don't want a Caesarean.
- Forceps are not to be used.
- I want the labor to last only five minutes.
- At the moment of birth, the suite is to be totally silent.
- While we're at it, I want one of those orgasm-labors rather than a painful one (see pages 151–152).

It is great that couples are well informed about the birthing process and the various options that may come into play. It is good that couples feel empowered and knowledgeable and that the husband (you) has some idea about your wife's preferences so that you can be her aide and advocate. But I also think that birth plans can be problematic.

A birth plan commodifies childbirth into a list of options, like the boxes on a hotel breakfast menu. But, unlike your nursery decor, a birth is a lot more complex and you can't pick and choose to any great degree what is going to happen when the baby comes out. You can pick a birth like you can pick the weather on your wedding day.

Also, when births don't go according to plan (and they often don't), many couples get disappointed – some bitterly – that the whole shebang wasn't what they ordered. Many things can happen in the delivery room, from a medical emergency to some advised intervention from your midwife or doctor. The laboring mother may have a change of mind about birth position or pain relief. If and when this happens, there's no point saying, "Hang on a second – let's consult the plan!" It is in fact more common to hear the woman scream, "SCREW THE PLAN! I don't care what you do, just GET IT OUT OF ME!"

Birth plans can be a hindrance rather than a help to medical professionals. Aside from it being slightly presumptuous and insulting (what other profession invites clients to turn up with a five-page list of conditions?), it can also cross the line into "precious" territory. As an example, take the following demand to an obstetrician from an online birth-plan generator: "If I have to have a C-section, please respect my wishes for quiet during the operation (e.g., avoiding 'small talk' with other practitioners in the room)." Really?

Some online birth-plan generators punch out a complex list of multiple pages covering every stage, decision and eventuality. Once things are underway, you can't expect the professionals to be leafing through Page 4, Appendix B, Sub-Section 2, searching for your whims on whose voice the baby will hear first after being born or the degree to which you want to be consulted about your baby being given eye-drops. Again . . . *really*?

So how do you strike a balance between a custom-designed birth, where you decide everything, and having no say at all in the birth?

Be well informed. Learn about it and know your options. Discuss these as a couple and with your obstetrician or midwife. Have preferences and hopes, but be flexible. While Meredith was not keen on the idea of having an epidural, I certainly would not have discouraged her if she grabbed me by the throat and screamed for one in the delivery room. As it turned out, she didn't have any pain relief for any of her three births. (She is a better woman than me, Gunga Din, 'cause I would have opted for them all in the first ten minutes.)

And if the doctor said to me, "Dr. Downey, I'm going to have to do an emergency Caesarean section," I wouldn't have said, "Hang on, doctor, just let me consult our plan."

If you absolutely feel you must have a birth plan, fine. But let it be no longer than this one I found on a blog: "Dear Midwife, please do whatever it takes to help this baby be born and for me and my baby to be healthy." Yay for common sense.

The aspects that you might need to be flexible with on the spur of the moment include the following:

Induction or Augmentation

If labor hasn't started or is going too slowly, the staff may contemplate and start talking to you about whether or not to "induce" or "augment" the process.

Induction is an artificial triggering of labor when it doesn't start naturally. This may be because there is a concern with either the mother or the baby, or, as was the case with us for Rachael, the baby is late. Induction tends to be considered when a pregnancy goes into its 42nd week.

Induction can be done *chemically*, through an oxytocin or Syntocinon drip, or by introducing prostaglandin to the cervix. ("Mrs. Cervix, this is Mr. Prostaglandin. He's just moved here from the Seminal Vesicle and doesn't know anyone. I'm sure you'll get along just fine. Can I offer you an hors d'oeuvre?")

It can be done *manually* by separating the membranes from the womb or rupturing the membrane inside the uterus with a long hook, causing the water to break. This uncomfortable but speedy procedure is called an amniotomy, and the hook is called "the hook."

Cervical thinning and opening can also be encouraged *mechanically*, using the delightfully named Cook Cervical Ripening Balloon. This is a double-headed balloon catheter that is (somewhat painfully) inserted and placed at each end of the cervix, and then is inflated with small amounts of saline to gently pressure the cervix into opening.

Some people fly the flag of more au naturel methods, including a brisk walk, a good swim, herbal tea, castor oil, or eating pineapple or a bowl of vindaloo. I suspect we are heading into old wives' tale territory with all of these, and, besides, does a pregnant woman really want the gastro-intestinal side effects that often come with the last three?

Stimulation of the nipples is often mentioned as an effective technique – hers, that is, not yours – because it triggers the release of the oxytocin hormone, which encourages labor. I don't know if it actually helped Meredith, but it sure helped me. Sex is also said to trigger labor, as semen naturally contains the hormone prostaglandin which encourages contractions. Sex with a nine-months pregnant woman is interesting, to say the least, but hopefully for her it's more fun than having a drip or an injection.

Augmentation is simply a booster to the process that has already started naturally but is moving a little too slowly. Either way, this is an artificial means of telling the body to "Get on with it!" This may involve therapeutic rest, drugs, oxytocin, anaesthetic, changes of position or a delivery assisted by instruments (see below).

Pain-Relief Options

Let's not dick about. With the exception of the rare orgasm-birthers (!), childbirth for most women is, essentially, painful.

And it is important to acknowledge that everyone has their own pain threshold. At one extreme is the mom who calls for an epidural at the first contraction, while on the other is the mom whose body is being split open by a Kaiju emerging from her vagino-portal, and she just bares her teeth and says, "Bring it."

If the pain of childbirth is too much to bear, you can stick your fingers in your ears and think of a happy place. But, while this might help *you* cope with the pain of childbirth, it won't be of much use to your wife. There are many options and techniques that laboring women use to help them power through the childbirth experience and surf the pain-wave. Many women report that a proactive approach and lots of preparation and exercise help them to feel in control during the birth. They say that facing up to, and "owning," the pain (rather than pretending it won't be there) helps them feel determined, resilient and confident about what lies ahead, rather than being a sad victim of circumstance.

During birth class, they will practice various breathing techniques and vocalizing (sound and movement exercises such as thigh slapping, fist clenching, chanting, rocking, etc.) that will assist them to manage the pain. Yoga and/or prayer can also be helpful in preparing the mind and muscles for the demands of birth.

Birth class will also cover various birthing positions, because – as mentioned previously – the on-your-back-with-feet-in-stirrups position is great for TV but terrible for childbirth. Ultimately, a laboring mother will find her own position of most comfort. For many, it is on all fours, in a bean chair, a semi-crouch or reclining in water. An upright squatting position allows the mother to shift about to accommodate the movements of the baby as it emerges from her body, and also allows gravity to assist.

The mind is said to be the most powerful tool in dealing with pain, so some women report success with hypnotherapy, prayer or meditation as ways of relaxing and reducing their fears around childbirth. Visualizing is also encouraged. This is where, instead of thinking about *the pain the pain the pain,* the mother focuses on the outcome and purpose of the pain, namely *the baby the baby the baby.* She visualizes dilation and the baby emerging through the birth canal, or other happy thoughts such as pinning you against a wall and punching your head in because you're the bastard who got her there in the first place.

You can also help her by massaging, applying hot packs, holding her in the best position (you in a headlock), whispering encouraging words ("You're doing great," or "I love you," or "If I could swap places with you, I would" – but let's be honest, that would be a lie) or playing relaxing music (FYI: a midwife let me into Secret Midwife's Business that they are sick of hearing anything Gaelic (#Enya) or with birdsong or waterfall noises).

Even with all these options, sometimes the pain is too much and your wife might decide she wants drugs to help her cope. A subtle hint that she has reached this conclusion is when she puts her hands around your throat and screams into your face, "PAIN RELIEF – *NOW!*"

Most women use *some* form of pain-relief drug during birth. Stats show that in most states, 60 percent or more women opt for epidural or spinal anesthesia. This figure varies between regions and depends on the age of the mother; asking why New Mexico is 22 percent and Kentucky is 78 percent is an interesting conversation starter guaranteed to get you uninvited from dinner parties.

When I say "stats" above, by the way, I'm not just making it up. All percentage statistics in this "To Plan or Not to Plan" section are from the National Vital Statistics Reports, the CDC, and the American Society of Anesthesiologists. They are indicative averages only, representing a wide spread of regional differences.

In terms of pain relief, hospitals have come a long way since the flask of whisky or bullet to bite. One option is a TENS machine, much like the one your physical therapist uses on you after you jam your back during an ill-advised game of football against your nephews at a family-reunion picnic. As the full version of its name suggests, it provides transcutaneous electrical nerve stimulation through pads placed on the skin.

Another option is a combination of nitrous oxide and oxygen – laughing gas – just like the stuff you get at the dentist's. It dulls the pain and makes it feel like someone else is experiencing it in the next room. Only 1 percent of women in America try it, but it's more common abroad. While the gas is safe for both mother and baby (because it is quickly expelled from the body), it has variable impact. Works well for some; not for others. If you're quick, you might be able to get a few lungfuls yourself.

An intramuscular (IM) narcotic injection – morphine – is a stronger form of pain relief, an opiate that relaxes the mother and alters her perception of the pain. It is usually not used in the later stages of the labor because it may affect the baby's breathing. Some women don't like this option because it can make them drowsy and nauseous, and they lose some sensation and don't fully "experience" the birth – which is ironically why other women like it.

The slam-dunk option is the epidural, utilized by about 60 percent of all laboring mothers (although the rates in some areas are more than double that in others). This is when a local anaesthetic is injected via a catheter into the woman's spine, which knocks out the lower half of her body. She doesn't feel a thing but remains awake to witness the event, which is probably like watching someone else give birth (even though her angle of vision would be quite unique). Again, some women don't like the idea of an epidural for this very reason. Also, it restricts movement and the woman's ability to push, and significantly increases the need for instrumental assistance as well as worse perineal tearing (see below).

It is important that you read up on the pros and cons of pain-relief options and discuss them with your obstetrician or midwife prior to the labor.

Breech Birth

Generally, babies are born head-first. This is so they can see where they're going on the way out. About one in thirty, however, don't get into that position at full term, and so they try to come out bum or feet first.

This is called a breech birth. (This is not to be confused with the word "breach," as in Shakespeare's play where Henry V encourages his followers to go "Once more unto the breach, dear friends.")

Traditional practice has seen, as a cautionary measure, almost all breech babies born by the surgical intervention known as Caesarean birth or C-section (see below), although there are reports of a recent shift in thinking around this, suggesting a normal vaginal birth for breech babies can be offered in certain circumstances and situations.

Tearing and Episiotomies

The basic physics of childbirth are that something relatively big (baby's head and body following) has to pass through something relatively small (cervix/vagina). These openings stretch to accommodate the passage of the newborn, and when I say stretch, I really do mean *stre-e-e-etch*.

For about a quarter of birthing mothers, this stretching, although painful, takes place without incident. Everything stretches, the baby is born, it shrinks back and all is well. This is known as that biological region being "intact." Over 50 percent of birthing mothers, though, experience grazing or tearing. This is mostly a slight loss or split of skin (and, in half of these cases, the tearing of the pelvic-floor muscle as well), which will usually require stitches. In very rare cases, it can be what is classified as a fourth-degree tear, where skin, muscle and tissues split back to the anus. Obviously, addressing this is a significant medical procedure.

Take a moment until your eyes stop watering before reading on.

An episiotomy is a surgical operation where the woman's vaginal opening is anaesthetized and cut to make it bigger and easier for the baby to pass through. This used to be a lot more common and standard than it is now, because both research and anecdotal evidence is pretty conclusive that in terms of invasiveness, recovery and healing, natural tearing is preferable to an episiotomy. An episiotomy is only performed now when necessary, perhaps because the baby is in distress or a complicated situation has arisen such as their shoulders refusing to deliver through the pubic joint. Ask your medical professional under what circumstances an episiotomy might be considered.

Caesarean Birth

This is where, rather than the baby being born naturally, it is removed surgically; essentially, it is cut out of the mother. This process used to involve a vertical cut from the mother's throat down to her knee, but advanced medical technology means that a modern Caesarean is only a small horizontal cut along her bikini line. The cut may look small, but, because it is quite invasive, the mother can't do anything too strenuous for several weeks afterwards. In fact, a full recovery from a Caesarean takes about a year.

Recent years have seen a massive rise globally in the rates of Caesarean births, and in America Caesareans represent about a third of all births. There is a range of arguments put forward as to why this is so, depending on who you listen to and what drum they are banging: mothers are older; doctors are worried about litigation; mothers are more overweight; doctors have become more medically conservative; celebrity mothers have popularized the C-section; a Caesarean can be scheduled and managed more easily than a lengthy vaginal birth; private hospitals jump to Caesarean births too quickly; the polar ice caps are melting . . .

Sometimes, this procedure is an "emergency C-section," meaning that it wasn't planned. Once labor is underway, there could be an unforeseen complication with the birth (and there are plenty to choose from) or a developing issue with either the mother or baby during labor that presents an increased risk to their health. Fortunately, despite the word "emergency," it is rarely the panicked spectacle of TV-drama births, where the surgeon yells out, "We gotta go C-section – NOW!" and everybody in the delivery suite starts running around shouting "STAT! STAT!"

Statistically more likely is an "elective Caesarean," which means the surgery is planned ahead of time. Contrary to popular belief, elective Caesareans are not the domain of SUV-driving, latte-sipping, future soccer moms in private hospitals (nicknamed the "too posh to push" set) who simply don't want to go through the ordeal of birth and want to preserve their pelvic floor. Despite a lot of noise about "maternal request" C-sections, there's usually a medical reason for the decision.

Either way, unless it's done under a general anaesthetic, most hospitals allow you to be with your wife during the operation. You have to gown up and you are only allowed near your wife's head, there to provide assurance. You don't get down on the business side of the screen to pass the surgeon scalpels and gauze.

The rising incidence of Caesarean births is a concern to many in the childbirth profession. They see it as negation of the fact that the woman's body is designed to give birth. It is a natural process, not something foreign that has been inflicted upon her, like a disease to be avoided. Then again, that's easy for me to write. I'm a guy and don't have to face up to the whole thing myself.

Again, the important thing is that you and your wife are well informed about any risks and advantages of a C-section. Make sure you ask your medical professional about their approach and experience in relation to Caesarean birth. (Some obstetricians and hospitals have high statistics in this regard and a reputation for promoting and defaulting to the Caesarean very quickly.)

My mother had a complicated pregnancy and, as a result, I was a Caesarean baby. That's why I have a big head and have trouble finding hats that fit me.

Baby-Removing Devices

Sometimes, in the middle of a delivery, the baby gets cold feet and decides not to come out. Like an overweight spelunker, it can get stuck in the claustrophobic confines of the birth canal. If it is well and truly wedged, or in distress, or if exhaustion or the anaesthetic have rendered the mother's pushing ineffective, there are two main devices that can be used to remove it:

- *Forceps.* These gigantic barbecue tongs are used to grab the baby's head and pull it out (the whole baby that is, not just the head).
- *Ventouse.* Think of a vacuum cleaner with a toilet-plunger attachment on the end. You will be pleased to know that this is purpose-built and there is little risk of your baby being sucked inside out.

Both of these options may cause some alarming markings or bruising on your baby's face and skull, where the device has got traction. Don't be concerned. They clear up after a few days.

Incubator or Humidicrib

Most babies have a "normal birth" and adjust to the outside world very quickly. Some, however, can have complications and need to be monitored closely. This can be the case with premature babies, low-birth-weight babies, babies with severe jaundice, babies with breathing irregularities and some Caesarean babies.

If your baby comes into one of these categories, it might be placed in a sealed crib, or incubator, which is hooked up to lots of machines that go "beep" and "ping." These machines help to monitor your baby's bodily functions, including body temperature, breathing and possibly feeding as well. Many parents feel intimidated by all the tubes, gauges and flashing lights. They may also find the incubator frustrating because they are physically separated from their baby by a plastic shield. But you can still touch your baby through portholes, and spend time sitting next to it and talking to it. Often, normal feeding is possible as well.

Ask the staff questions about your baby and the incubator. The staff in special-care nurseries are accustomed to anxious parents and will help you to feel more comfortable about the situation. In any case, remember that your baby won't be in there for too long.

What's in a Name?

It is a truth universally acknowledged that the single biggest cause of marital disputes in Western society is the choice of names for an impending child. While finding a name that *you* like is pretty hard, finding a name that you and your wife *both* like is next to impossible.

Because it may take a lot of time and many nights chewing over your options, you should do your research and start working through potential names well before your baby is born. This gives you both plenty of time to fight about it.

Some influencing factors could be:

- *Family tradition.* Our Georgia scored her name because of lots of Georges on both sides of our families, while Rachael got her grandmother's middle name, Emily.
- *Religious reasons.* Some people may want to name their children after a notable historical person within their religion, perhaps because of their character, deeds or teachings: Hannah, Sarah, Noah, Luke, Joshua, Muhammad

. . . although it's probably best to stay away from Rahab, Judas or Maher-Shalal-Hash-Baz.

- *Meaning.* While some parents couldn't care less, others think the meaning behind a name is important, such as Peter (rock) or Meredith (protector of the sea), also avoiding others such as Mallory (unfortunate) or Claude (cripple). This is where a bit of research, on the internet or from those curiously titled "Baby Name" books, pays off.

- *Nationality.* As above, this is more important to some parents than others, but many names can be traced back to their countries of origin. Parents might be from a particular country which is an important part of their identity (Ferdinand? Hilda? Theo? Campbell? Jacqueline?), or they might simply like that country or its perceived characteristics.

- *Character.* Stemming from Puritan religious traditions are names that themselves declare an admirable characteristic or trait: Hope, Faith, Joy, Felicity and Prudence, for example, although you'd want to stay away from their more extreme examples, such as Humiliation or Calamity. Also, you want to hope that they will live up to their name and it doesn't instead become an ironically incorrect moniker: Chastity or Grace, for example.

- *Musicality.* Some name combinations just sound right and have an appealing rhythm to them. I like the name January Jones.

- *Or it could just be simply because you like it.* Matilda got Ellen as a middle name, which I have liked ever since I saw Sigourney Weaver play Ellen Ripley in the *Alien* movie franchise (Meredith wouldn't let me call her Ripley). If aliens ever come to Earth, our Matilda will be able to stand against them.

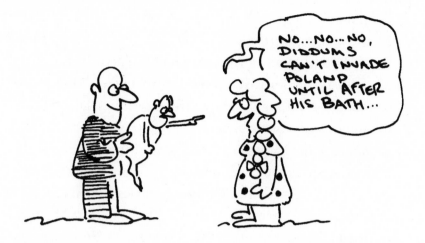

There are also a few names that parents might want to think twice about:

- *"One-off" names already belonging to a famous person or character.* It's their name; let them have it: Frodo, Elvis, Azaria, Madonna, Tarzan, Hamlet, Cher, Noddy, Voldemort, Bono, Sting, Goofy, Enya, Santa, Tupac, Homer, Oprah, Beyonce, The Artist Formerly Known as Prince, Darth, Moby, Pink, Usher, Gotye, Katniss.
- *Bad persons of history.* For obvious reasons: Idi, Adolf, Benito, Lucifer, Attila, Imelda, Ghengis, Lucretia, Saddam, Osama, Kony.
- *Crazy celebrity names.* These names are kind of edgy and cool, but a little bit pretentious if you're just an ordinary kid in the suburbs among the Ryans and the Nikkis: River, Storm, Leaf, Shade, Thorn, Park, Moon Unit, Stone, Rock, Branch, Ocean, Cotton, Apple, Peaches, North West, Pilot Inspektor, Moxie Crimefighter, Flea.
- *"Unique" spelling names.* Some people are condemned to have to spell out their name every time they speak it throughout

their entire lives, and have it perpetually incorrect on school reports, certificates and official documents: from the traditional Siobhan (pronounced Sh–ugh–vorn) through to ordinary names that parents try to make sound more cosmopolitan through slightly variant spellings, generally in the unnecessary introduction of a "y" (Jaymes or Olivya), a redundant double letter (Maxx or Kenn), or by replacing one letter with another to create an eyebrow–raising variant (Amelia becomes Akelia, Virginia becomes Virlinia).

- *Unfortunate first name/surname combos.* The actor Rob Morrow named his daughter "Tu." (Wait for it . . .) Enough said. (My Aunty Ida Downey also fell victim to this carelessness on the part of her parents.)
- *Any names that appear in songs.* These include, but are not limited to: Roxanne, Sharona, Lola, Fernando, Dolly, Ziggy, G–l–o–r–i–a, Eleanor Rigby, Jake the Peg, Barbara Ann, Eileen, Jude, Billie Jean, Proud Mary, Mustang Sally.

Then again, if you follow my advice above, you will name your child Karen, Kathy, Jane, Lisa, Peter, David, John or Michael, like the nice kids in an old novel where they discover smugglers down at the cove.

Another problem is that even when you *do* agree on a name, as soon as the baby is born you will look at it and realize that the name is wrong.

"He just doesn't look like a *Porl*," you will say.

Then you have to start all over again.

To Cut or Not to Cut?

Circumcision is the surgical removal of the foreskin off the penis.

The removal of a little bit of skin doesn't sound like much, does it? . . . But let me tell you, if you want to ruin a dinner party, mentioning the idea of cutting off the tip of your son's diddly-o-tiddle-whacker is just the ticket. (Closely followed by vaccination, but more on that later.)

Circumcision has been around since Year Zero. In different communities, it is significant for reasons of health, hygiene, appearance or religious observance.

Look, I've got no particular drum to bang and no experience to draw from (#onlydaughters), but, for what it's worth, here's my view. If all is fine (and aside from religious observance), I don't think boys should be circumcised. "But I was circumcised, damn it, and it didn't do me any harm!" I hear you cry. "Why shouldn't I have my boy 'done'?" According to my wife, it's because circumcision is cruel, unnecessary and has no medical justification. I have less noble reasons.

When I was born, circumcision was standard practice and as such I received the big cut as a matter of medical course. It was "the done thing." I don't remember how I felt about it at the time, but twelve years later I was quite happy, because I "looked the same" as all the other naked boys in my high-school locker room. Having a different organ in this situation meant suffering the worst taunts.

In 2012, the American Academy of Pediatrics found that the health benefits of newborn male circumcision outweighed the risks of the procedure. However, the benefits aren't significant enough for the organization to recommend universal newborn circumcision, and the AAP says that the final choice should still be up to parents to make based on their own beliefs. Health experts keep debating whether circumcision is a good idea.

The circumcision rate in newborns has been declining in recent decades, though most American boys are still circumcised. For a lot of parents, it comes down to appearance: they want their son to look the same as his family and friends (not to mention, the other guys in the high school locker room); no one wants their son to be the odd one out. But with many parents choosing not to circumcise, who's to say what "normal" looks like?

If you need help making the decision, talk to your doctor. But know that there's still a debate over whether the procedure is necessary or not.

To Jab or Not to Jab?

Talkback radio and the internet are frequently the forums for fiery debates about immunization, with both camps offering passionate arguments for and against. You and your wife should discuss which side you're on before the birth of your child.

Let me remind you that, although I have a First Aid Certificate and am called Doctor, I am in no way a medical expert. Having said that, I think immunization is a good idea – a view, I might add, that is held widely by the global medical profession and the World Health Organization. I have no desire to risk my kids getting polio, bacterial meningitis, whooping cough, measles, mumps, tetanus, rubella, diphtheria, bubonic plague, human papillomavirus, halitosis or dyslexia.

Most kids in America are immunized. It takes place at regular intervals, largely when your baby is between two and eighteen months of age, with a few boosters in adolescence. Don't get swayed by emotional arguments or oddball blogs, forceful opinions or herd mentality. Rather, look at the hard data relating to the risks and benefits of immunization. Talk to your doctor and plow through some reputable websites.

When You Least Expect it

The countdown is almost at an end . . . the due date. Your research is complete. Family and friends are primed and on alert. The nursery is furnished and ready for operation. You've been to classes, chosen possible names, read the books, scoured the websites . . . Your wife's bag is packed and sitting by the front door. Your miscellaneous digital devices are charged. The car is fuelled and pointed in the direction of the hospital. You've played the whole thing out in your head in those sleepless moments. Bitten your fingernails. Bought the Moët. All you need now is for the star of the show to arrive.

Problem is . . . despite your best efforts, your baby doesn't know or care about your schedule. It will come out when it damn well feels like it.

You can't spend the final weeks following your wife around on the off chance that she might start having contractions. When Meredith was in her final weeks with our first daughter, Rachael, I must admit to being something of a concerned – some would say even obsessive-paranoid – father-to-be.

I remember coming home from work one day during her "final week."

The house was empty.

Clearly, Meredith had been rushed to the hospital by ambulance, where she was giving birth at that very moment.

I freaked out and phoned the hospital: "Hi. My wife's pregnant and her name's Meredith and she's not home. She's having a baby and I just got home and my name's Peter and she's not here and she's due this week. Her name's Meredith and we're having a baby. Did I mention that? She's pregnant. My name is Peter. Is she in the labor ward? Is it a boy or a girl? This *is* the hospital, isn't it?"

The nurse on the line did her professional best not to sound too patronizing or annoyed, but I could tell she was busy and thought I was an idiot.

"She's not here. She's probably shopping. Goodbye," was all she said.

She was right. Meredith was shopping. I was an idiot.

Make sure your phone is on whatever setting will get your attention. Then, the only thing left to do is wait.

Wait.

Wait.

Because, any second now, my friend, you'll get a call, or a nudge, or a curiously exaggerated eyebrow lift accompanied by stomach clutchage (I made that word up) . . . and, at that moment, everything you thought you knew about life will come to an end.

Oh yeah. On my signal . . . unleash hell.

6

A Good Day
for a Birth

"When you do actually go to the hospital, *don't* wear good
shoes. They'll only get ruined."

A Brief History of Labor

Over the course of history, labor has changed.

In her classic *Clan of the Cave Bear* stories, Jean M. Auel
describes life at the dawn of time. When the pregnant woman
felt her first contraction, she was exiled to a dark corner
of the cave with other women to writhe through the agony
of childbirth on a mastodon-skin rug. Meanwhile, the "mate"
and future father sat with the men of the tribe around the fire
to discuss the day's hunt. The men knew instinctively that
labor was a "woman thing" and that this was not to inter-
rupt their evening men-of-the-tribe chat around the fire.

Many hours later, after all the action, the newborn would be presented to dad, who would grunt, scratch himself a few times, and pass the kid back.

He was definitely not a modern man.

Well, times may have changed but some things never do. The dark and smelly cave has been replaced by a bright and smelly hospital. The ochre paintings of bison on the cave wall have been replaced by pastels and flower arrangements in the waiting room. But, up until just recently, the inherent sexism of the labor process had pretty much remained with us.

It wasn't that long ago that men were still nowhere to be seen near a birth. You're probably familiar with the television-sitcom stereotype of labor. I was brought up on this and was almost disappointed when I discovered that it wasn't like that anymore. You know what I'm talking about? Four or five dads-to-be, eyes bleary from hours of coffee, anxiously pacing the waiting-room floor, eagerly expecting the door to open and the midwife to stick in her grinning head and announce, "Dr. Downey, it's a [insert appropriately] boy/girl/not sure yet!" I would then receive pats on the back while handing out cigars to all my paternal comrades.

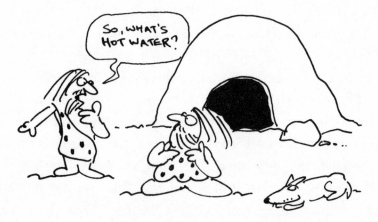

It doesn't sound too much different from the cave, does it? Fortunately, times have changed sufficiently that we dads now have an important role to play in the labor process. No longer do we have to wait by the fire in the cave. No longer do we have to wait in the waiting room. Now, we get to participate. We are there. Point-blank. 3D. High-def. Surround sound. The whole bit. And this is lucky for us, because being present at and participating in the birth of your child is a really wonderful experience.

Terrifying, yes. But wonderful.

However, you are not there just to spectate and take photos (see below). You are there for one reason, and one reason only. Be single-minded and clear on this: you are there to support your wife. You are there to soothe her, to encourage her, to reassure her, to hold her. To do this, you must be totally focused on her needs and on the labor.

Should I Be at the Birth?
Yep.

But, What's it Like?
Before we go further, I want to make one point clear: childbirth is *painful*. It may well be a natural and normal part of a woman's biological journey, but it is still painful. Very, *very* painful.

That bit in Genesis in the Bible was not off the mark where it says, "With pain you will give birth to children."

Sure, this is not always the case. Apparently, there *are* women who genuinely don't feel any pain with childbirth, or who feel only mild discomfort. Some have even described it as physical pleasure. I used to think this was a childbirth urban myth, but the YouTube clips of women who had orgasms during birth would appear to prove me wrong.

Yes, you read right: orgasms. (Don't get your hopes up. This is rare and odds are on this will *not* be your wife.)

There is nothing in a man's natural lifespan that even comes close to the agony that accompanies a baby tearing itself from its mother and being squeezed out into the world . . . although I have heard strong counter-arguments from sufferers of kidney stones or guys who weren't paying close enough attention when in the vicinity of a wood-chipper.

Unfortunately, we have fallen victim to pathetically unrealistic television portrayals of labor. These portray labor as little more effort than a light aerobics session. The hapless woman pants a few times, blows a few breaths through clenched teeth and then, with a Herculean push and a final gasp, gives birth to the baby in the UTBP. (Check out the ridiculous birth scene in *What to Expect When You're Expecting*, when a woman pops a baby out during a sneeze.)

This is crap. Total and utter crap. Childbirth, on the whole, is painful.

Just imagine trying to urinate, um . . . a lemon. Get the idea? (For those offended by this analogy, yes, I understand that the urinary and reproductive systems are different. That's why it's an *analogy*.)

When Meredith was first pregnant, I played her a motivational talk by some southern business guru. At one point the guy says, in a thick drawl, "With thuh burth of mah furst chahld, my wahf and ah had uh paaynless layburr."

Meredith didn't think this was very funny.

I'm sure it was painless . . . *for him*. Although I'm not a medical giant, as a veteran of three births now it's fairly safe for me to claim that, generally speaking, childbirth is not painful for us men. (That is, unless you have extreme

Couvade syndrome (sympathy pains), or you're a traditional Huichol Indian male who attaches a rope to his scotum for his laboring partner to yank upon during contractions, just so *he* knows what it feels like. So the story goes . . .)

Here's how I came to an awareness of the pain of child-birth. Soon after I found out that Meredith and I were going to be parents, I became quite inquisitive and anxious about the whole labor process. And then, one day, at an afternoon tea, we met an old friend who had just had a baby. What a perfect opportunity! Unashamedly, and in retrospect stupidly, I opened our conversation by asking her, "So hey, is, um, childbirth painful?"

There was a brief moment before the corner of her mouth curled up and her eyes narrowed. Fixing me in her steely gaze, she said, "Imagine you are holding an umbrella."

Mmmm, okay so far, I thought.

"Now," she said, pausing for dramatic effect, "insert it into your penis."

I crossed my legs and tried to break eye contact, but she held me in her gaze and pushed on mercilessly.

"Now open the umbrella," she hissed.

With alarm bells clanging in my head, I staggered to my feet in a feeble attempt to escape my groinal anguish. But I wasn't fast enough. She grabbed my arm and snarled in my ear, "Now pull it out. Yank it – hard."

She was revelling in the paralizing effect of her words.

"That's what childbirth is like," she snickered as I hobbled off.

Lights . . . Camera . . . Action!

We live in a highly visual era where the taking and sharing of photos and videos is part of daily life. Given that many people make a habit of snapping and sharing pics of even the most mundane guff – like the meal they're about to eat or the sunset outside their window – something much more momentous such as, say, the birth of a child, is bound to warrant some photographic attention. Fair enough. But how far are you going to go with this photo thing? How many photos are you going to take, and of what? What will you video? And, more importantly, what are you going to do with those images?

Here are my five rules about taking photos/videos during the birth.

Rule One: Discuss it with Your Wife Beforehand

This is the most important rule of all. During labor, your wife will be in no state to direct the photography. So discuss beforehand what she wants or permits you to photograph.

My anecdotal vibe is that most women want no photos of the birth itself. Aside from modesty issues, they want to be in the moment, and not distracted by photography. They're happy for a few tasteful snapshots before labor really kicks in and after the baby is born. (Besides, what do you do with birth photos anyway?)

Rule Two: Discuss it with the Medical Personnel Beforehand

As a courtesy, you should raise the question of taking photos and videos with your obstetrician or midwife and ask about their attitudes in different potential situations. It is likely that they will not have any objections at all about you taking still photographs. However, you cannot assume that they will allow unrestricted video. In the United States, and in some Australian hospitals, an anxiety about litigation has caused the introduction of restrictions, or even bans, on filming. This is especially so in the case of a Caesarean birth (either planned or emergency), or during a birth where unexpected complications arise.

Rule Three: Remember Your Role

Keep in mind that you are by your wife's side during the birth to do one thing: provide support. Don't be fooling around with your camera or phone when your wife needs words of assurance or simply your company, support and attention. You're not going to be much use to anyone perched in a corner trying to delete pics from your last vacation from your phone to free up some memory.

In addition, you certainly don't want to antagonize her with unreasonable photographic requests, such as:

- "Hey, that was great – can you make that face again?"
- "Now . . . you take one of me standing over by this monitor here."
- "Can you lift your legs just a *bit* higher?"
- "Don't push . . . I have to recharge!"

Rule Four: Don't Get in the Way

The midwife, obstetrician, your wife and, when it's born, the baby don't want to be blinded by constant explosions of light from a camera flash. It may be wise, therefore, to adjust your settings so your photography can be unobtrusive.

If you want to shoot video during the birth (and it's permitted), that's your business, but stay out of the way. Medical personnel may not mind if you set a camera rolling in the corner, but you can expect opposition if you keep trying to play with the GoPro you've strapped to your wife's inner thigh.

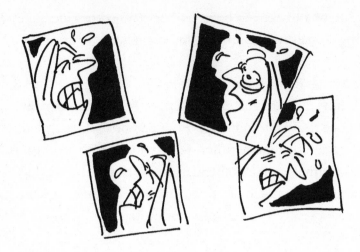

Rule Five: Don't Get Carried Away

The excitement of the moment may impair your judgement about what is appropriate to share online with friends. While you might be quite moved by the awe of the birth, your friends, family and colleagues won't appreciate receiving footage of "placenta being delivered" while they're having their breakfast.

Resist the temptation to Instagram (or whatever photo-sharing app is popular at this moment) in some kind of pseudo real-time coverage of the birth event. If you want to share photos, do it later, after you've calmed down a bit.

Zero Hour

The phone rings. Or she nudges you.

Okay, this is it. Zero hour.

The final grain of sand has fallen through the nine-month hourglass and it is time for the baby to come out into the real world. There are early-warning signs that it's all about to go down. One signal is a "show" (technical name: *operculum*, if you must know), which is a euphemism for the expulsion of a sticky glob of mucus that has been blocking up your wife's cervix for the past nine months, to prevent the entry of bacteria. It may also be signalled by the delightful euphemism of when "the water breaks." This is where the uterine cocoon ruptures and all the amniotic fluid spills out like a scene from *The Dam Busters*. (Great fun if you're at a restaurant or in a traffic jam!) Or it may be signalled by the commencement of regular contractions, which is when your wife's uterine muscles get together in waves of tensing and relaxing in preparation for the Herculean task of pushing the baby out. This is the beginning of the first stage of labor.

Contractions are described generally as intense period pain (a useless description for us guys) or extreme abdominal and back cramps. (Maybe think medicine ball and testicles?) Coming in waves, they can start mild and far apart but increase in intensity and frequency in preparation for the birth. By the time they really kick in, they are an all-encompassing pain that would stop a buffalo in its tracks. One of your jobs is to time and record these contractions, as this is important information for hospital staff to get a read on where the labor's at.

You need to record how long each contraction lasts (its *duration*) and the gap between each contraction (its *frequency*, timed from the start of one contraction to the next). Due to my OCD nature, coupled with new-dad-birth-anxiety, when Meredith's contractions started, I commenced a rigorous recording regime across several bits of paper, including the occasional hastily scribbled graph, for illustrative purposes. I found these tremendously interesting and reassuring. My long-suffering wife, however, did not. Fortunately, there is now a range of simple contraction-counter apps and websites that will do all the work for you with the click of a button.

I always assumed that Meredith's contractions would kick in at about 2 am, several days before the predicted date. I imagined scrambling for the car keys in pajamas and slippers and making a dash to the hospital in the freezing dead of night. Of course, contractions can come at any time, and their onset certainly does not mean that the baby is about to be born within minutes. Some people find that labor can be a very lengthy, and consequently exhausting and frustrating, process.

This frustration can be even worse if your wife has a false labor. The contractions kick in, everybody gets psyched up and you go to the hospital, but after a while it becomes apparent that nothing is going to happen, and the nurses send you home. Your wife's body was playing a practical joke on her! These premature contractions are called Braxton Hicks contractions, and are the uterus's way of practicing for the strong contractions needed during labor. (I pity the crazily bearded Dr. John Braxton Hicks, who named these contractions in the 1870s, leading to centuries of women cursing his name.)

It is also frustrating when the baby is late. Most first-time mothers will have their babies on average about eight days after the due date. It is hard not to subconsciously psych yourself up for that date, and you may be anxious if you've arranged your work schedule around that time. But then the big day passes. The next day passes too. And the next. And the next after that. And then, after that, the next day passes. Finally, the day after arrives and then unceremoniously passes as well. The expectation and tension increase until you're a nervous wreck. This is not helped by well-meaning people at work who each day ask, "So, the baby hasn't come yet?"

("No, Sherlock.') It's like *Groundhog Day*, where every day seems exactly like the last. Basically, you just have to grin and bear it. *Que sera, sera* . . .

We were pretty lucky with the births of our babies. For our first child, Rachael, I woke up on a Friday morning ready to go to work after a good night's sleep and was confronted by my wife saying, "Okay, I think this is it." It was a beautiful summer's day. The sun was shining through the window and the birds were singing as we had breakfast. Rachael was born just after 11 am. She was two weeks late.

For our second child, Georgia, we were just clearing the table after a very pleasant dinner when once again Meredith said, "Okay, I think this is it." Georgia was born close to midnight. She was one day late.

For our third, the Tillster, I was sure we could get it right on the day − just to confuse our obstetrician. But then we traveled down the familiar road of one day, two days, three days late. Then, on the fourth day, right in the middle of *The Simpsons*, Meredith said with great certainty, "This is it." Matilda was born a few hours later − twenty minutes off being an April Fool. Phew.

The point is that "it" can come anywhere, anytime. It could be midnight or midday. You might be in bed or on a train or at a dinner party or driving a plow. (As a matter of fact, it could be now.) But when the time comes, there's no point saying, "Can you just hang on a minute?" You must be ready. The bomb is about to go off.

There is one important thing to remember at this moment. In the immortal words of *The Hitchhiker's Guide to the Galaxy*, **DON'T PANIC**. Even if it is an emergency situation (i.e., the baby's head is sticking out), remain calm and in control. Do not, for example, run around screaming, "What do we do? What do we do?" Do not run for the car semi-naked from your interrupted shower with shampoo in your eyes.

This is where all your careful planning pays off. If you are having a home birth, start running the bath. Boil some water and tear up a sheet into strips. (I'm not sure why, but that's what they always did in old movies.)

If you are going to the birth center or hospital, give them a phone call. They'll probably ask you a few questions about whether there have been any discharges (water breaking, the show, etc.) and they'll also want to know about the frequency and duration of the contractions, and tell you when they think you should come in. They certainly don't want you coming in too early, because this makes the whole process more drawn out and could even delay the birth because the stress of the change of environment can disrupt the labor. Going in too early also means that if the labor doesn't progress, you get sent home, which is frustrating.

Most people make it to the hospital on time, but some don't. They might get stuck in traffic, their car might break down, or the birth may strike sooner than anyone could have predicted. If it is an emergency situation, again, **DON'T PANIC**. Remember, childbirth is a *natural and normal* thing. It has been going on ever since Eve said to Adam, "Okay, I think this is it." Three hundred babies are born every minute in the world, most without the luxury of freeways and hospitals, so you're certainly not doing anything new. A woman's body is designed for childbirth. It is a fully automated process.

Statistically, it is highly unlikely that you won't make it to the hospital. But, on the off chance, there is a protocol to observe. If you're in the car, pull over somewhere safe. Don't stop in the middle of an intersection or outside a boys' high school during their lunchbreak. If you're in a taxi, make sure the driver turns the meter off. If you can, get someone to call an ambulance.

Then do your support stuff, just like normal. Don't freak out. Your wife will need you more than ever before, and your panicking won't make things any easier for her. Help her to find her best birthing position, then get down near the baby-chute and catch it as it comes. Let the goop come out of its mouth. Wrap the baby up in a sweater or towel to keep it warm. Don't pull on the umbilical cord or cut it; the placenta will come out by itself. Then go directly to the hospital. Do not pass GO and do not collect two hundred dollars.

Then put your car up for sale for half its market value.

One final word of advice: if and when you actually get to the hospital, *don't* wear good shoes. They'll only get ruined.

Stage One: Before Birth

Birthing still retains a certain sense of mystique in our society. Some people liked being born so much that they go to "rebirthing clinics" to try to experience the whole thing all over again. Some states even have a public holiday to commemorate the wonder of the birthing process. This is called Labor Day.

In any discussion of childbirth, it is necessary to talk in generalizations because every pregnancy and every birth is unique, and some are even bizarre. For example:

- Gorgias of Epirus was born in his mother's coffin during her funeral.
- In 2012, twins Amy and Katie Elliott were born eighty-seven days apart.

- There are several recorded cases of twins being born having different skin color.
- A baby was once born to a virgin. This was about two thousand years ago and the case received a lot of publicity. A lot of people around the world are still interested in this birth.
- In 1875, a seventeen-year-old girl became pregnant after a bullet fired in the nearby Battle of Raymond lodged into her uterine wall. She didn't know that the bullet had already carried off part of a soldier's left testicle. Nine months later, she gave birth to an eight-pound boy who had to be operated on to have the bullet removed. The soldier and the girl later married. (Interestingly, the TV show *Mythbusters* tackled this story in 2005, and "busted" it. Um, okay then.)

Trying to cover every eventuality, situation and circumstance of birth would be impossible, but here's a general overview of a typical hospital birth.

Okay. You're driving to the hospital. Despite what they do on TV, don't run red lights at full speed or drive up on the pavement, scattering cafe diners. (Having said that, I always harbored a secret fantasy of getting pulled over by the police and then getting an escort (with sirens and flashing lights) to the hospital.) Remember, don't panic. The worst thing you can do is drive erratically or dangerously.

You arrive at the hospital. Grab someone wearing a uniform and tell them what's going on. (Make sure it's a medical-looking uniform and that they are not a cleaner or caterer.) You will have already filled out forms and things a while ago, and as you've probably already phoned they'll be expecting you anyway. Eventually, you will be shown to a labor ward or delivery suite, where the hard part begins.

The wait.

Your wife may have a quick labor: You arrive at the hospital. The baby is born. The end. (Unlikely.)

Or your wife may have a long labor: You arrive at the hospital. You hang around for ages getting exhausted, frustrated, sore and hungry. The baby is born. The end. (If you are mixing in "new parent" circles, you have no doubt already heard the horror stories.)

While acknowledging a very broad scale of experience, the average time for the first stage of labor is in the ballpark of ten to twelve hours. During this time, the contractions build in intensity. They get stronger, closer together and longer in duration. By the time of birth, the uterus has grown to be the biggest and strongest muscle in your wife's body, so you can imagine the strain this puts on her as the contractions increase.

Meanwhile, you are waiting for the cervix – the passageway out of the uterus – to get bigger. The cervix has for the past nine months essentially been the gatekeeper at the bottom of the uterus, keeping the baby in and other stuff out. But now it has to open up or "dilate" until it is big enough for the baby to pass through. Some people refer to this process as "waiting for the cervix to ripen," which in my mind conjures up awful images of rotten fruit. But that's another story.

The cervix looks kind of like tiny pouty lips and is quite hard, like cartilage, but as birth approaches, it begins to dilate, where it softens and stretches to a diameter of about ten centimeters to allow for the transition of the baby's head.

From time to time, a nurse might pop in and give your wife an internal examination to check the degree of dilation and progress of the baby. After the first cervix inspection, the nurse will probably say, "Two centimeters," which is code for, "You'd be lucky to give birth to a walnut right now."

Fifteen minutes later, when your wife has experienced so much pain that she is sure a school bus could drive through her cervix, the nurse will come back, inspect, and say, "Three centimeters." The nurse will then go and phone your obstetrician and tell him/her how many more rounds of golf could probably be fitted in before needing to get to the hospital.

If your wife is not able to swallow fluids, she might be kept hydrated with an intravenous saline drip. In addition, a synthetic hormone such as Syntocinon may be administered, which helps encourage the uterus to get on with the job of contractions. When Georgia was born, I asked the midwife for a bourbon drip but she didn't even crack a smile. Maybe she'd had a long shift?

So, labor can be long, painful, tiring and frustrating for mothers, many of whom by this stage are starting to have second thoughts about their babies and just want to go home and have a camomile tea. Once you see your wife going through contractions, you will agree that there is no doubt the female of the species really drew the short straw as far as childbirth was concerned. And so, the following comments are made in that context.

For both your own wellbeing and your capacity to be a great support to your wife, it is important you are prepared for the effects that the labor will have on *you*. Sure, you're not the one with the contractions, but you can't just stand back unaffected in the shadows either.

Childbirth for fathers is *draining*. It can be mentally taxing to focus on your wife for hours on end. It is also physically demanding. You might have a sore back and be on your feet the whole time, and you might not have eaten or had anything to drink for ages. It may be particularly difficult if your wife has labored through the night and you've both been awake for over twenty-four hours straight.

Because it's probably the first time you've witnessed child-birth (YouTube meanderings aside), it can also be *disorienting*. You'll be in a strange and perhaps sterile place full of machines that look like they belong in a nuclear missile silo. Medical personnel will come and go and sometimes talk about things you won't understand, so you can feel a bit disconnected, like you're in the middle of a whirlwind. You might not be really sure that everything is going as it should for your wife, and on top of that you may be anxious that the baby will be okay.

The experience can also be *harrowing*. It is not easy seeing the woman you love in so much pain. She will look at you with either pleading or accusing eyes and, aside from the aforementioned massages and assistance and words of encour-agement, there's not a great deal you can do about it. It won't be pleasant watching her struggle through it. Prepare yourself to be strong for her, and remember that all mothers you know – young or old – have gone through this before. It is a natural and normal part of life around the world.

On the positive side, however, childbirth is a *thrilling* exper-ience. It is awesome, in a genuinely gobsmacking way, to see your child come into the world. It is not uncommon for dad hormones to kick into gear and for you to feel a burst of love and pride and joy about your new family. It can be very emotional to finally meet the fruit of your loins and realize, "I'M A DAD!!!!"

As your wife nears the second stage of labor – the actual birth – she may appear increasingly vague. There will be a blank expression on her face and her comments may become more monosyllabic. Her breathing will change. All this is because a naturally produced opiate, endorphin, has entered her bloodstream. In short, she is stoned. She will internalize her thoughts, getting further away from reality. Her body, meanwhile, will experience waves of pain (or pleasure, as per previous) as the contractions get stronger and her cervix opens wider.

Throughout this entire process, remember your job: *you are there to help.* Don't let your mind wander. Focus. Encourage and support your wife. Hold her hand. Rub her back. Hum her a tune. Talk to her. Reassure her. Give her a sip of water. Wipe her face with a washcloth. Support her. Stroke her hair. Help her move around. Help her maintain a comfortable position. Tell her you love her and that she's doing great. If she is in the bath, pour water over her back. Let her get you in a headlock. In short, do whatever she wants if it will make her feel better.

Of course, this is assuming that you can actually *understand* what she is saying in the first place. Women in labor have a special, secret language, incomprehensible to the male ear. For example, she may point at the ceiling and say, "Grumph . . . hoooo . . . hoooo. Shup . . . den . . . plissss," and give you "the eye." Good luck trying to work that one out.

When she was having Matilda, Meredith slowly twisted her arm up and pointed behind her back. She muttered, "Harumph . . . sheejh . . . carrrmooon. Hhooo . . . hhrruuufffff."

I took this to mean, "Rub my back, just . . . there," which I did. Later, I found out she actually meant, "Whatever you do, don't touch my back here."

Just do your best.

Another thing you can do to help is encourage her to use the breathing techniques and exercises you practiced in your birth-education classes. Breathe with her and coach her through the contractions. Remain calm and controlled. Be relaxing. Say positive things in warm and whispery tones, such as:

- That's it . . . good . . . b-r-e-a-t-h-e d-e-e-p . . . b-r-e-a-t-h-e d-e-e-p . . .
- You're doing great. You're doing great.
- Almost over now.
- Relax, relax, relax.
- You are strong.
- Open, open, open, baby, baby, baby.
- I can see the baby's head.

Avoid saying negative things such as:

- Jeez, that's a lot of blood!
- Boy! I'm glad I'm not you right now!
- Hey, is that normal?
- I don't think this baby's ever going to be born!
- Is there anything in the fridge for dinner?
- STOP BEING SO TENSE!
- Oh, Toto, I want to go back to Kansas.

Once upon a time, women were supposed to be quiet and dainty while giving birth. But this is an unreasonable expectation. By way of illustration, try this exercise:

1. Put your hand on a solid surface.
2. Hit it with a hammer.
3. Stand still and make no noise.

I bet you can't do it, assuming you're not one of those psychopathic villains in action films who hold their hand over a blowtorch without flinching to show how tough they are. If you've ever actually hit yourself like that, you know you scream, moan, stomp, swear, yell, pace back and forth, jump up and down, and so on.

"Noise and action" is a popular childbirth pastime. Encourage your wife to make whatever noises she feels like and to move however she wants to if it will help her cope. This could be rocking back and forth, swaying, slapping her hands on her legs, moaning, repeating words, pulling faces, breathing strongly and steadily, and panting. Don't stand back snapping off photos of her behaving strangely. Join in with her.

About now, it is not uncommon for even the most meek woman to unleash a vitriolic string of swear words, some that you didn't even know existed, maybe even towards you. She is not being crude. There is significant academic research that indicates that (for people who don't swear much normally), swearing helps reduce pain. Which you perhaps already intuitively knew, as per the last time you sent your little toe into a door post. Normally sedate women may scream abuse and say things to their husbands they don't really mean, such as "I hate you for doing this to me," "I never want to see you again," "You're not really the father," and "Let's have another baby straight away."

As the second stage of labor approaches, the urge to push may become irresistible for your wife. Things are about to get a bit wild. Your baby is coming.

Drum roll . . .

Stage Two: Birth

This is when your baby is actually born. It can last from a few minutes to a few hours.

Now, let us for a moment consider how the baby feels about being born. For the past nine months, it has been happily floating in its own little world that it has come to call home. It spends its days sucking its thumb, dreaming and practicing for its black-belt exam. It probably really likes it in there. It's warm and the food is plentiful. If it had its way, it would not come out until it was eighteen years old, thereby avoiding school and many awkward moments during adolescence.

Then, all of a sudden, things turn sour. The nice warm fluid drains out and the baby finds itself inexorably pushed downward towards an impossibly small hole as if caught in some sort of vaginal tractor beam.

As you can imagine, it might not be happy about this turn of events.

For this reason, the midwife or obstetrician may decide to keep an eye on the state of the baby on its journey. This is done with abdominal dopplers (two bands around the mother's abdomen; one for contractions and one for the baby's heartbeat). These will monitor the contractions and let everyone know whether the baby is "in distress" or not, or if any torpedoes are coming towards you. If your wife has had an epidural, she will almost definitely be wired for sound, because she won't be able to feel the contractions herself.

Meanwhile, the baby's head will be slowly negotiating the cervix and making its way through the pelvis. If there is a problem with the size of the passageway, an episiotomy may be performed, or forceps or the ventouse might be brought into play to help. (Also, in large hospitals and with private obstetricians, it is routine to give the mother an injection to assist in delivering the placenta and to reduce bleeding later on.)

At this stage, after much "labor" from your wife, the head of the baby will pop out and turn around. Tension, noise, expectation. There may be a short pause. Then, with the next contraction, the shoulders will emerge, and finally the rest of its body. Smells, sounds, relief. It will shoot out into the world in a flurry of blood, mucus and a wash of unidentifiable, technicolor fluids of varying consistencies.

Ta-daaa!

And there in that moment right there, your life just took a ninety-degree turn, because . . . you, my friend, are now a dad.

Take a few breaths. Savour the moment.

Kiss your wife. Tell her she did good.

Look at the face of your child.

Snap off a couple of tasteful photos.

If you want to cry, do it. You wouldn't be the first.

One day, you'll look back and laugh.

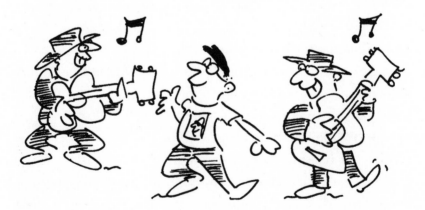

Stage Three: After the Birth

If the baby passed thick meconium (hideously sticky green early-infant poo, the result of ingesting fluid from the amniotic sac) before birth and it is clogging its mouth, it may be suctioned out. This is done by one of the nurses or the obstetrician by inserting a tube into the baby's throat and sucking it all out – an activity, I might add, that is never mentioned by nurses on Careers Night at school. With good reason.

The baby's reflexes will kick in and it will take its first breath. It will then be put straight onto mom's stomach for some warmth, skin to skin contact and a cuddle (even while waiting for the placenta or having stitches done). This is a special moment for the mother, where they finally get to meet the person who's been growing inside them for the past months.

At first, you may be surprised by how your baby looks. It might not be what you expected. This is because in commercials, on TV and in films, all "newborn" babies are in fact photogenic eight-month-olds who have just had their hair shampooed. Most have had acting lessons. Real newborns aren't like this. They are wrinkly little things covered in mucky, tomatoey gunk. They are also coated in a thick, creamy covering, called vernix, that looks like French onion dip. (Unlike babies in movies who are born like this but miraculously clean up within a minute or two, your baby will stay mucky for at least twenty-four hours.) They are usually squashed and have weird-shaped heads, and they may have bruises or marks from the tight squeeze, or from a forceps or ventouse extraction. Some are born with jaundice, which gives them a yellowish tinge, or a fine covering of body hair, called lanugo, which gives them a sort of werewolf look.

In short, newborn babies are ugly and messy. All of my kids looked like Yoda when they were born. But they're beautiful now. Really.

Another shocking and little-discussed feature of newborns is . . . well, how can I put this nicely? Um . . . you see . . . they have REALLY BIG GENITALS. Newborn boys are surprisingly well endowed, and girls' parts can be quite swollen. Both boys and girls can secrete milk from their nipples. But before you get too proud of the fact that your newborn son looks like some superhuman sex god, his scrotum, which currently reaches to his knees, will get small again after a while.

You will also notice that your baby is still attached to your wife by a long, thick strand of witchetty grub – the umbilical cord – that for months has supplied its nutrients and carried away its waste. But it can't stay dangling out of mom forever. This would make for many awkward moments, like, for example, high-school graduation. So the cord has to be cut.

Traditionally, the cord has been cut fairly quickly – in the first minute after delivery – although recent research suggests that there are benefits to waiting just a bit longer, while the placenta fulfills its dying duty of pumping the last of its goodie nutrients into the baby. (Ask your medical professional about their thoughts and practices on this matter.)

The dad is often invited to perform the momentous "cutting of the cord," which involves the highly technical process of the cord being clamped with big pegs while the dad squeezes a pair of scissors through the veiny thread. Some people ascribe great symbolism and significance to this. I totally get that, because it is that precise moment that your child becomes an independent *Homo sapiens*. I cut the cord of each of my children, although, to be honest, at the time I really wasn't that fussed about it and I was generally tired and felt slightly weird doing it. (Not a fan of blood, surgery, or organs.) I was more interested in my wife and the newborn itself.

When Rachael was born, I thought I cut the cord in the wrong spot, because her new belly-button was about seven centimeters long, like a squidge of penne pasta sticking out of her stomach. It's supposed to be like that. In the next few weeks, the cord will dry out and drop off by itself. Keep it clean and dry, and resist the temptation to tug on it. If you're lucky, you will find the shrivelled remnant in your baby's cradle or clothing and can have it bronzed and mounted to use as a paperweight.

Even after your baby is born, your wife has not yet finished her task. The placenta – your baby's life-support mechanism for the past months – is still inside your wife and has to come out. This is colloquially referred to as the afterbirth, because . . . well, it's self-evident, isn't it? Soon after the baby is born, the placenta will detach from the uterus and be "delivered" the same way. When it arrives, looking like a giant, hollowed, roma tomato, the placenta will be inspected to ensure it is intact, or whether in detaching itself it has torn, leaving remnants inside. If there are "retained products of conception," they are removed either by a firm rub on the mother's fundus (uterus) or by a trip to surgery for a "manual removal," where the doctor gives the mother a decent anaesthetic and then enters the uterus either with their hand or a large spoon-like implement to clear it out.

If you're lucky, the doctor will present the placenta to you and show you interesting things about it. At this stage, your wife might have to have some stitches if tearing has occurred, or if she has had an episiotomy.

Anyway, enough of this eye-watering stuff. If you are so inclined, and if you ask nicely, the hospital staff might let you take the afterbirth home with you. It sounds weird, but some people do. I know a couple who went to their friends' place for a morning tea. It was a nice morning, with tea and cakes and pleasant company. Then the hosts, who had recently become parents, whipped out a shovel and a suspicious-looking plastic bag and invited everybody down to the backyard for an afterbirth-planting ceremony. Not really my thing. Then again, it's better than being invited around for a placenta smoothie. (I'm not kidding, by the way. If you don't believe me, check out the variety of "placenta recipes" online, which will detail how to serve placenta on pizza, or as a roast, lasagna, soup, bolognaise, stew, or even a cocktail.) Again, not really my thing.

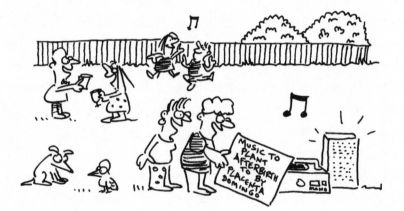

In the Silence

When the afterbirth has been delivered, most of the show is over. Equipment will be wheeled away. Some of the staff disappear. The mess is cleaned up. A strange quiet will fall over the room. The newborn is encouraged to have its first feed at the breast. This is an important moment of connection for mother and child.

For the first few days, the baby will receive a super-powered drink from its mother's breasts: colostrum. As it can sometimes have a golden hue, it is sometimes described as "liquid gold." It is thicker and stickier than more mature milk, which will kick in a few days later. Colostrum is an amazing cocktail, more powerful and potent than anything that could be dreamt up in a chemistry lab.

It is a turbo charge for the baby, a concentrated power drink that does several things. It has a laxative effect, to give the baby's new digestive system the kick-off it needs. It has a nourishing effect, as it is chock full of goodness in the form of, among other things, antibodies, amino acids, minerals, sodium, potassium, and vitamins A and E. And, importantly, it has an effect on the baby's immune system. Colostrum is full of immunoglobins, so it protects the baby from the nasties in its new environment, outside the protective confines of the womb. Colostrum is so good and beneficial that bovine (cow) colostrum is widely available as a dietary supplement shake taken by some athletes.

The midwife or doctor will do a quick assessment to check the health of your baby. This is done by a simple rating called an Apgar score, which looks at its skin color, breathing, reflexes, heart rate and muscle tone. (Apgar is not an acronym but is named after the grandmotherly and bespectacled Dr. Virginia Apgar, a twentieth-century anaesthesiologist who devised the test.) FYI, a score of 3 or below is potentially critically low and a score of 7 or above is normal.

The baby may also undergo a quick and simple hearing test. It will be weighed, and the diameter of its head may be measured. While it's your choice, it has been standard procedure since the 1980s for babies to receive a vitamin K injection immediately after birth. The American Academy of Pediatrics has recommended this since 1961. This helps their blood to clot and prevents bleeding disorders. Speak to your midwife or obstetrician about this beforehand.

A hospital tag will be attached to the baby's wrist detailing its name, weight and time of birth. This is to avoid confusion and prevent parents from fighting over whose baby is whose later on.

Your wife might have the opportunity to have a wash or even take a shower, but she'll probably need your assistance.

And that's about it.

The baby will be put in a nightie and wrapped up tightly in a blanket. Then the staff will probably leave the three of you alone to get to know each other.

After the noise, pain and turmoil of the birth, it's really nice just to relax and enjoy your first moments alone together in the silence. After nine months of waiting, there is a certain sense of awe and wonder in seeing your baby for the first time. You will notice little things, such as its fingers and toes, eyes and ears, and the folds of its skin. This whole experience can cause an adrenalin rush that will leave you on full power for the next few sleepless days.

And, as the three of you sit there exhausted in the delivery room, you may start to think, "Phew, thank goodness that's all over."

Heh, heh. It's only just beginning.

Bonding

You have probably heard of this thing called "bonding," which is the process of being bound, fastened or held together, like your fingers, if you've ever tried to superglue anything. More than that, it is something that unites individual people and connects them in a special relationship. This word is thrown around quite a lot in birthing circles. It refers to the process by which you feel joined to your baby; when you feel that "it" is part of your family; when you feel an emotional involvement; a link that unites you both; a feeling you have that *you are mine*.

There's a general vibe around baby circles that bonding is instantaneous and absolute, kind of like in the movie *Avatar* how the Na'vi warriors bond with their flying mountain banshees using their hairy ponytail things. While not always the case, bonding with a newborn appears to be more of a natural and intuitive process for mothers, perhaps because they have already been carrying the baby inside them for months or because of the hormones released during childbirth or during breastfeeding.

But it's not necessarily as automatic for dads.

I expected this bonding to occur the moment our baby popped out into the world.

It didn't.

I expected to look at it and experience a warm glow of love and attachment.

I didn't.

I expected it to be magical, mystical and instantaneous.

It wasn't.

When my kids were born, it was pretty amazing and all that. But I didn't feel "bonded." I wanted to. But I was tired and a bit disoriented. I was wondering where the violins and soft focus were. Meredith, on the other hand, bonded straight away. As soon as our baby was in her arms and feeding, she was off with the pixies. She was stroking skin and looking at her baby with a deep of look of contentment, love and adoration.

To be honest, it took me quite a long time to bond with my children. Sure, I felt a little flutter when I held my own child for the first time or when a little hand squeezed my finger. But I wasn't, well, ga-ga. My head was tellin' me, "This baby is yours; it is part of you and your wife." But my heart was tellin" me, "Sorry, who is this stranger?"

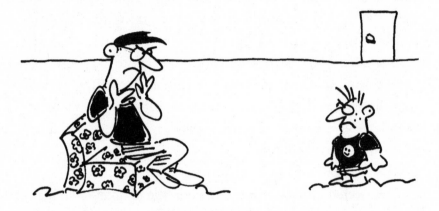

Looking back, there were many moments over the next weeks and even months when I felt this "bonding" thing occurring: a long, sleepy cuddle in the afternoon sun; the first time Rachael's eyes followed me; the first time she smiled on seeing me; the first time she reached for me; the first time she fell asleep on me; the first time we went to the store together with her slung in a pouch; the first time she vomited on me; the first time she said "Daddaddadda" – at least, that's what I think she said.

In retrospect, I realize my expectations were as out of whack as expecting to love Meredith the first moment I saw her (even though I must admit I was mighty attracted – oh yes I was). Bonding is a relationship thing, and any social-theory textbook will tell you that a rich relationship or even a feeling of attachment doesn't occur at a snap of the fingers. It takes time.

Like most experiences in becoming a dad, everybody is different. I know of some guys who really did bond instantaneously. They picked up their newborn and almost swooned. The coming days were spent totally obsessed with this new addition to their family. These are the guys who Instagram eight different photos of their baby's feet taken from different angles.

I know others who, like me, were fairly nonchalant at first towards their newborns but warmed up after a few weeks.

Don't be stressed about bonding. It'll happen when it happens.

Celebrating

Well, congratulations. You can now officially call yourself a dad. Welcome to the WWF: not the World Wrestling Federation but the Wonderful World of Fatherhood.

Such a monumental step as this is cause for a monumental celebration.

As a child who grew up on TV sitcoms and cheesy movies, I was always entranced by the depiction of proud dads celebrating the birth of their first child with their friends. This largely involved drinking champagne, making a lot of noise and, most importantly, smoking cigars. And come rain, hail or shine, I knew that this was what I was going to do when my first child was born.

And so Rachael arrived. I was so charged up after the birth that I didn't sleep for a few days. Everything fell into a kind of timeless, euphoric haze, which had started off with a great celebratory get-together. I invited a bunch of friends around to our place to watch gripping selections from the hours of video I had shot. Everyone congratulated me on the great job I had done. What an achievement! I could be proud of myself! That night, the el-champagno did flow, and my pals and I went through a box of cigars. This is ironic considering the only thing that I detest more than champagne is smoke. But this was what had been programmed into my mind by years of sitcoms, so champagne and cigars it would be!

Meanwhile, my wife was lying exhausted in a hospital bed, trying to cope with the demands of a new baby. When I came down and hit "the wall," not only did I feel physically exhausted and lousy, I also felt guilty that I had let her down like that. Perhaps I would have been better saving my strength and spending a bit more time at the hospital? Perhaps I should have postponed my celebration until both my wife and our baby could also attend? After all, they were the stars of the show who did all the hard work. All I did was lose a piece of my scalp to a woman who chose to go without pain relief.

I had learned my lesson. When Georgia was born, the celebrations were a lot more controlled. I had a light beer and a pencil-thin cigar and only stayed up for forty-eight hours. And when Matilda was born, I finally got it right. I celebrated with a kebab and a peppermint tea, and went to bed early . . . and lay awake all night.

Take it Easy

It is very easy to get excited about the birth of your first child. Even if you haven't quite bonded in a personal way, there is still a great sense of occasion, and you are still riding the momentum of nine months of expectation. You feel like you have jet lag, and time loses its meaning. After all, it *is* a pretty big deal, and your family and friends make you the center of the universe for a brief moment. And, after witnessing the miracle of birth, it's little wonder you get emotionally carried away with the whole thing.

However, it's easy to lose your perspective and begin to think that the birth of your child is the single most momentous event of the century. This is called paternal tunnel vision (#PTV).

The first signs of this syndrome are excessive photographing, videoing and social-media updating. Because everything is so new, and it's such an important event, you want to capture as much as possible for posterity. I, for example, became an obsessive photographer of hands and yawns.

(The main problem, as any parent with two or more children will tell you, is that the first child scores their own pregnancy–birth blog, a huge canvas wall poster hung over the dining-room table and a cute YouTube clip with an inspiring soundtrack that you secretly hope will go viral. The second child appears in a status update on your Facebook page, gets a framed photo on your bookshelf and a well-meant but ultimately unrealized intention on your part to send a selection of photos to your family. The third child ends up with a lone tweet and some hastily snapped and blurry photos that never make it out of your phone.)

Another symptom of PTV is an inability to talk about any subject other than your baby. You should take care to avoid lengthy monologues with neighbors, friends, relatives or colleagues regarding fatherhood. Remember that while your life has been turned upside down, their lives have gone on as normal. Most will want to know how the birth went and how mother and baby are doing, but they don't want to watch a collection of little clips on your phone of "us having breakfast on the morning of the birth," "a quick tour of the maternity wing and miscellaneous interviews with interesting people I met there," "mother and baby minutes after birth," "floral arrangements in the labor room," "me talking to camera as I drive home from the hospital," and so on.

As per the original "pregnancy announcement," social media is a quick and convenient way to spread the good news to large groups of friends and family. It's more time-efficient than contacting everyone individually, albeit less personal. Again, though, make sure you get personally in touch with the key players in your life first. Your mother-in-law doesn't want to receive a retweeted proclamation that your baby has been born (#helltopay). Remember to keep it simple, and that less is more. People want to know the baby's name and weight, time and date of birth, how mom is doing and how it all went in brief. They want to see a photo or two of the new arrival.

If you go to the bar for a celebratory beer with your work-mates, they too probably don't want to discuss the ethics of intervention in birthing; they don't care about torn perineums; they don't want to debate the advantages of breastfeeding over bottle feeding; and they won't be interested in updates on the progress of baby fecal consistency.

There is also common decency to consider. Some things are supposed to be kept private. I'm not sure your wife would appreciate you narrating graphic descriptions of her torn vagina or cracked nipples. My wife certainly didn't.

She's Got the Blues

I had heard about this thing called the blues, the period of moody sadness suffered by some women following the birth of their babies. But I knew that it wouldn't happen to my wife. The blues were for *other* women; women who were emotionally weak or prone to depression. Soft, weepy, frail women. My wife, on the other hand, is just about the most level-headed, down-to-earth and fully-in-control person you are likely to meet. So the blues didn't apply to her, right?

Wrong. During the last weeks of pregnancy and particularly during the labor itself, women overdose on their naturally produced opiate, endorphin. After the birth, most women have enough hormones pumping through their veins to knock down an enraged bull elephant at twenty paces. But then the opiate dries up and they go cold turkey. Added to this is the fact that childbirth is painful and physically demanding – women do not recover overnight, particularly if their labor was long, traumatic or if they had to have stitches or other interventions. The whole situation is exacerbated by altered sleep patterns (read: "lack of sleep" patterns) and the repetitive demands of a continuous stream of visitors. There is also the nervous anxiety and mental pressure of being responsible for a new and fairly demanding human being. The result is a potent emotional cocktail known as the blues.

Depending on your source, somewhere around seventy to eighty percent of women experience the baby blues, in their first couple of weeks after birth. This is why, when you visit a maternity ward, somewhere in the distance you can always hear the twang of a steel guitar, the wail of a harmonica and a chorus of mournful female voices singing:

I had a baby the other day
And I can hardly walk
My nipples are dry and cracked real bad

And my husband and I don't talk
I got the blues
I said I got those moody bloo-oo-ues
I got the baby-makin' breastfeedin' down 'n' out maternity blues.

All women will react differently, but the blues can be triggered by almost anything and usually manifest themselves in mood swings and spontaneous crying. You can't argue with it or talk your wife out of it. Your job is to help and support her in the most appropriate way possible. Be sensitive and understanding. Encourage her. Comfort her. Talk to her. Hug her. Be there for her and the baby as much as possible. She needs rest, so help out by taking the baby or by managing the onslaught of visitors (see below).

Don't tell her about all your troubles at work. Don't tell her about all the great parties you've been going to. Don't tell her she's being silly and that she should grow up and stop crying like a little girl.

Put your arms around her, damn it!

For most women, after a couple of weeks the hormones will settle down and the off-kilter ship will right itself and everyone will settle in to the routine of a new domestic life.

For some women (about fifteen percent), however, the blues don't go away. They just get worse. This is a serious condition known as postpartum depression. Sufferers can feel lost and confused, tired and miserable, like they are in a black hole from which there is no escape. The whole routine of domestic life with a baby dulls their senses, and simple tasks and chores take on overwhelming proportions. Things are made worse if there are problems with breastfeeding. They may have trouble bonding with the baby and difficulty making decisions. They may also feel emotionally on edge and as though they are isolated from real life, and swing between feelings of low worth, anger, anxiety, isolation or helplessness. These feelings may manifest in physical ways too, such as loss of appetite, tiredness and lethargy (which are perfectly reasonable when looking after a new baby). In extreme cases, there could even be thoughts of self-harm or harm to the baby.

Postpartum depression can last for months. Be open to discussing this with your wife. Support her, encourage her and spend time with her. Provide her with adult conversation. Tell her not to feel guilty or ashamed of her emotions. Help to organize the domestic routines and provide stability and order around the home. If appropriate, arrange friends or relatives to visit her. Find out about local groups with which she can become involved and connected, such as mothers' groups, playgroups, Bible studies and online communities. But, most importantly of all, seek professional counselling. Call your hospital, doctor, midwife or local baby-health or early-childhood center for more information. There are loads of online and telephone support groups and organizations that can provide support and assistance, as well as many self-test-type questionnaires that can help you to understand what she is going through.

Whatever you do, don't ignore it or pretend it will go away. Again, if things start getting bad, seek professional assistance.

It is also worth noting that some men also experience depression as a result of becoming a new dad. While they don't have the hormonal changes throughout pregnancy or the physical trauma of labor, they can still be thrown by the crazy new world of fatherhood. Overwhelming feelings of responsibility, fear, inadequacy, changes to routine, lack of sleep, lack of sex, mourning the loss of the way things were, anger and disappointment can all contribute to a depressive malaise.

Again, it is important for you to know that this is "normal" and you would not be the first to be going through this. It is important for you to acknowledge that our culture is not necessarily very good at allowing or expecting men to feel or express emotion, and that old-school, "chin up, man up" attitudes will do nothing to help the situation. As per your wife, it is important for you to know it is okay to seek professional assistance and, for the good of you, your wife and baby, you should do so.

Guests

It's good to have friends. Of course, your friends and relatives will want to share with you and your wife in your new-found joy. Many will want to visit mother and child in the hospital, and bring gifts and ogle over and maybe even cuddle the baby.

Visitors are a good thing. They can break the monotony of the hospital or home routine for your wife and cheer her up if she's feeling down. It's great to see familiar faces, and a few flowers around the place certainly brighten things up. But visitors can become a real pain, the degree of which is mathematically correlated to the number of friends and relatives you have, the hours they choose to visit, the average length of time they stay, the volume of noise they generate, the number of photos they take and questions they ask, and how incapable they are of taking a hint that you want them to leave.

The main problem is that visitors are exhausting. If you're really unlucky, they will come in a constant stream, one after the other, like a prearranged tag-team, with an endless repetition of photos and questions and presents and chatter and laughter and noise . . . all day long. Mother and baby will end up wrung-out, stressed and irritated.

This is where you step up. Be aware of your wife's needs. Maybe she and the baby don't want visitors straight away? Maybe your wife is exhausted and needs a bit of time to recover? If this is the case, tell your friends to hold off for a few days, and then try scheduling them so they don't all arrive at once. Also, inform them of the assigned hospital visiting hours. This will ensure that both your wife and the baby get a decent rest. I have some friends who instated a two-week embargo on any visits at all (lifted for only the most immediate circle of family). They wanted to find their feet first and settle in back at home.

Also be alert to your wife's desire for privacy. This may come as a surprise to you, but she may feel slightly uncomfortable about whipping out an engorged bosom for breastfeeding in front of all your basketball teammates, particularly if baby is being uncooperative.

It's your job to run point and protect mother and child. Just because someone wants a cuddle of your baby doesn't mean that they can have one. Don't be afraid to say no. Don't let people have hot drinks near your baby. And watch out for grandmas wearing brooches on their shirt or jacket. My nan used to wear jagged, bejewelled brooches that looked like a ninja throwing star. You don't want your baby's face rubbing up against that. And don't ever be afraid to tell your visitors – no matter who they are – when it's time to leave. If they don't take the subtle hint, tell them you've got the placenta in a bag in the bedside table and you want to show it to them . . .

Get Ready – They're Coming Home

Soon, the time will come for your wife and baby to return home from the hospital. If you're smart, there are a few things you can do that will help this grand homecoming run a little more smoothly. The general household routine will be pretty tumultuous for the next couple of months while you both get used to living with and caring for a little person in the house, so use the brief time you have alone to make some final preparations. This will get things off to a good start.

Have the house clean and tidy and "ready for baby" on their return. Trust me when I say that family life will not get off on the right foot if your wife comes home to unmade beds, a pile of laundry, ironing, dirty dishes, dusty shelves, a pile of pizza boxes in the corner and an expectation that you've been waiting for her to come home so she can tidy it all up. Some balloons and flowers probably wouldn't go astray, either.

An empty fridge will also not endear you to your wife, so stock it. When Meredith was still in the hospital with Georgia, I went to the local butcher and bought bulk supplies of ready-made stir-fries and marinades. I spent one morning in the kitchen cooking them all up and dishing them into takeout containers. I labelled them and filled the freezer to overflowing. Why not fill up your fridge with pastas and sauces? Mixed with freshly cooked vegetables and rice, and interspersed with salad and the occasional takeout, these supplies lasted us many weeks and especially helped on those days when things were a little hectic. (I am talking about decent food here, not high-fat, high-salt cocktail franks, party pies or frozen pizzas.)

It is also important for you to get some sleep. If you are going to help out with the baby, you need to be rested and alert. All-night binges and TV marathons will just wear you down at a time when you need to be strong.

The Calm Before the Storm

Up to now, things have been kind of nice. You have probably been going to work and then popping into the hospital for the occasional visit. You've been able to hold your baby for a little while, spend a bit of "quality time" with your wife and then go back to the "real world." In fact, it's been almost like a holiday, living by yourself for the last few days. You could please yourself around the place, drink straight from the bottle, watch old sci-fi movies, sleep across the entire bed, leave the seat up and eat vindaloo. It's all been quiet and nice.

This is the calm before the storm.

Your baby won't stay in the hospital forever. After a few days, the staff will say, "Right, go home!" You pick up your wife, the baby, the bags, cards and flowers and head out. I had a strange sensation when we stepped across the threshold of the hospital door clutching Rachael. The electric doors zooshed closed behind us and I looked around and thought, "Really? Are you guys really just gonna let me walk out with this baby?" But no alarms went off, so we kept going.

The first thing you notice is that "the two of you" are now "the three of you." There is another human being in the back of the car.

This is where all your training and reading and discussion and contemplation get put to the test. This is where theory meets reality. Life will never be the same again. So strap yourself in and let the grand adventure begin.

You are about to encounter the storm after the calm.

7

There's a Baby in My House

"If you are an 'I mow the lawn and wash the car and the wife does the shopping, washing, tidying and cooking' kind of guy, then you'll need to rethink and retrain."

Life Beyond the Birth

Weddings are interesting.

People who are engaged spend a lot of time planning their "big day." For months and months – years, in some cases – their entire existence is directed at the thousands of intricate details that go into having one of those fairy-tale weddings like in the glossy magazines in your doctor's waiting room.

And so comes the great event. The wedding. After all that effort, everything goes smoothly. The wedding runs like clockwork and, in a flurry of rice and confetti, the bride and groom drive off into the sunset with a tremendous sigh of relief that it's all over.

Of course, it's not over at all. It's just begun. I think some couples spend so much time focusing on their wedding day that they forget to spare a thought for the much more important part beyond . . . their lives together. And so, for some, the early days of marriage are a shock to the system, like spending a lot of time organizing a flight overseas but not bothering to think too much about what you do once you clear customs in a distant country.

The same applies to having a baby. It's easy to spend all your time devoted to the "big day" of the birth – in books, conversations, birth classes, and so on – while neglecting to look beyond, to the more important part that is to follow . . . being parents and living with a new little person in your home.

This is a b–i–g mistake. It is vital that you and your wife spend time *before* the birth thinking about and discussing life *beyond* the birth.

The Times They Are a-Changin'

Take a breath and get a picture in your mind of what your life has been like, pre-baby.

Got it? Good.

Life with a newborn is not like that.

When our first child was born, one of the biggest surprises for me was that she was so . . . so . . . (how do I put this without sounding like an idiot?) . . . 24/7. Babies are very demanding of time, and the little time that they do leave you is necessary for sleep. As such, there are many elements of your domestic life that will have to adjust to your new situation. Here is a list of things that become difficult when you have a baby living in your house. Note that I said "difficult," not "impossible":

- listening to loud music
- listening to quiet music
- going shopping
- washing the dishes
- washing the car
- washing yourself
- washing clothes
- hanging out clothes
- ironing clothes
- mowing the lawn
- curling up with a good book
- watching a movie without interruption
- wasting hours watching inane YouTube clips
- having a relaxing evening together at home
- having an in-depth, adult conversation
- going out
- sleeping through the night
- sleeping in
- having sex on the spur of the moment
- having sex even if you plan it carefully
- even thinking about having sex
- updating your social-media profile
- cooking
- eating in peace
- cleaning the house
- practicing your musical instrument
- working at home
- writing a book.

In addition, your home will look different than how it looked before. You may have a spacious and airy home; a home built for entertaining; a home filled with interesting and beautiful things. You may have an obsession with tidiness and cleanliness.

All of this will have to be overcome.

For the next few years, your home will be a wasteland. Your windows will be smeared with greasy fingerprints. Grapes and bananas will be squashed into the carpet. There will be a constant smell of urine and ammonia, and every so often there'll be a hideous waft of something ghastly that you just can't locate. Every nook and cranny will become home to a million tiny building blocks, crusts, stuffed toys, little cars, broken crayons and dolls' clothing. All drawers and cupboards below the three-foot level will sooner or later have their contents strewn randomly throughout every room.

I wish I could say something like, "No, wait! Babies do actually make your life easier! You'll hardly notice they're there."

But that would be a lie.

Babies are lots of work. They are. That's the truth of it. Sure, it's great and all that. Being an active and involved dad, you need to share in that work. I don't know what your domestic situation is; whether your wife is going to be a full-time home-maker or go back to work after a while. It may even be that you are so emancipated that *you* will be the one to stay home and look after the baby. Or the economic reality of today may mean that you both work full-time, in which case a lot of thought needs to be put into daycare and job division. Whatever it is, though, you will need to discuss and plan your domestic duties and, once again, "get your hands dirty."

Of course, the work you do may not necessarily involve the baby directly. Regardless of what your domestic habits or roles have been in the past, if you are an "I mow the lawn and wash the car and the wife does the shopping, washing, tidying and cooking" kind of guy, then you'll need to rethink and retrain. And, whatever you do, never, ever, *ever* walk in the door and say, "Why is the house such a bloody mess? What's for dinner?" Old jungle saying: Never cross a tired woman with sore breasts.

Bosoms and Bottles

There will always be topics over which people will argue:

- Mac or PC?
- Jesus Christ: liar, lunatic or Lord?
- What *really* happened to Jimmy Hoffa?
- Who was the best James Bond: Connery, Moore, Dalton, Brosnan or Craig? (Oh, all right, or Lazenby?)

And this golden gem:

- Should a mother bottle feed or breastfeed?

The feeding of babies is a surprisingly contentious issue. Advocates of either method can become very fiery about their beliefs. The two enemy camps – The Bottle Alliance and United Breastfeeders – each have their own online communities, newsletters and surveillance satellites.

Given that so much shelf space in the bookstore parenting section and many million websites are dedicated to baby feeding, it would be ludicrous of me to attempt to go into detail about feeding options. But, just for the heck of it, here are the main arguments:

Breastfeeding:

- is natural
- uses "live" milk, full of antibodies that strengthen the baby's immune system
- encourages closeness and bonding between mother and child
- can split the mother's nipples
- can be awkward or inconvenient in public for some mothers (even though in this day and age it shouldn't be)
- can be frustrating and time-consuming
- can't be done by you, the guy
- can be affected by the mother's diet (onions, nicotine, garlic, etc.)
- can utilize bottle technology for babysitting purposes
- may make aspects of work or social life more difficult
- is cheap (free!).

Bottle (formula) feeding:

- is not done by any other mammal on the planet
- can be done by men
- is not "live" from the mother but is derived from cow's or soy milk and supplemented with various vitamins and minerals
- keeps the mother's nipples in one piece
- means messing around with bottle kits and sterilizers
- can give more flexibility in relation to work and social options
- is easy to prepare for babysitters
- is a genuine and viable alternative for women who are unable to breastfeed
- costs money.

I have a bias towards breastfeeding, for three reasons:

1. UNICEF (along with pretty much any medical organization on the planet) says "Breast is Best."
2. It makes intuitive sense.
3. My cousin is a lactation consultant and family gatherings will be intolerable if I don't fly the breastfeeding flag, so to speak.

It is generally considered that babies should be exclusively breast-fed for six months and then combo breastfed with the gradual introduction of solids up to between one and two years. Sure, there are some "earthy" parents who will claim that it's cool to breastfeed a child up to six years of age, but I'm not convinced. My personal litmus test is if the baby can operate an iPad, they are too old to breastfeed. If they are old enough to enunciate the words, "Mommy, my show has finished and it's time for booby," then it's time for them to get off the Glands of Montgomery.

Either way, your role is important. Newborns feed every few hours, twenty-four hours a day. This means getting up regularly throughout the night. If your wife breastfeeds, you can get the baby for her and put it back to bed. If your baby is being bottle-fed, you can assist with the workload.

You can also help by burping your baby. Because they guzzle and suck so greedily, babies often swallow air while feeding. This sits in their stomachs and causes them discomfort, which leads to crying, which in turn causes stress, tension and sleeplessness in their parents (see below).

To burp your baby, hold it upright with its head over your shoulder and gently pat its back while you hum a tune and sway back 'n' forth. After a while, the baby will come forth with a deafening peal of thunder – the kind of burp you'd expect to hear from a sumo wrestler. It is also usually accompanied by a hefty curdled-milk projectile spew, although this normally only happens when you've got a good shirt on. If you ever play rub-noses with your baby after they have had a feed, make sure your wife is videoing you, because then she can capture the moment when the baby projectiles into your mouth, and you can put it on YouTube.

If your wife decides breastfeeding is the way to go, fantastic. But if bottle feeding is your only option – if, say, your wife is sick or under stress, or if the baby is unwilling to go on her breast – that's fine too. Babies are nourished by formula everywhere in the world, every day of the year. So read some books, talk with your wife and discuss it with your doctor and the hospital lactation consultants to work out which option is best for your wife and your baby.

And two other things. I shouldn't need to say these, but I will . . . just in case:

1. Don't ever use breastmilk or formula in tea or coffee.
2. Some women lactate with only the slightest prompting. Never say to a breastfeeding mother stuff like, "Hey, so you're breastfeeding, huh? Wow, it's really physically intimate, isn't it? How amazing to have your own body giving nourishment to your child, to see the baby's mouth on your breast and to hear the *schloop schloop* noise as your milk flows. It must be a wonderfully satisfying sensation . . ." They will not be happy.

The Crying Game

Babies cry a lot. *Who knew?* I didn't. I think that is because, as a child, the only baby I ever saw was Jesus in nativity drawings on Christmas cards. Have you ever seen a Christmas card where Jesus is crying? No! He is always asleep. What a deception. (Actually, perhaps this in itself is actually proof that Jesus was the Son of God. But I'm sidetracking.)

We have a neighbor who has a faulty car alarm. It goes off at all hours of the day and night. *Wwwaaaaaeeeeerrrrr. Wwwaaaaaeeeeerrrrr.* It is an excruciating klaxon wail that goes on and on and on until all the people on my street are driven to the point of insanity. When it starts up, I feel like taking to his car with a hammer.

Imagine having a car alarm that lives in your own house. It goes off regularly during the day and night. And imagine that you have to pick the car alarm up and cuddle it and kiss it. You sing to it and mumble soothing words and, guess what, it just gets louder! That's what a baby in full cry mode is like.

Babies cry. That's their job. They're particularly good at it. In fact, some babies love to cry. And when they cry, they are not doing it because they want to sound nice. A baby's cry is most often loud, incessant and very irritating. That's what it's supposed to be like. It's an attention-getter. It says, "Hey, you, come here! I want something!"

When you or I want something, we go and get it. If we feel uncomfortable, we fix ourselves up. If we're thirsty, we go to the fridge. If we're hungry, we dial for pizza. However, babies can't do this. Their single form of communication is crying. So they'll cry if they are lonely, thirsty or hungry, if they are cold or hot, if they are tired or wet, if the TV is too loud or the light is too bright or they have a pain. They'll cry because it was nicer in the womb, or because they don't like the way you decorated their nursery.

In short, babies cry about just about anything. Of course, the problem with this is that all creatures great and small have an instinctive protective response to the crying of their offspring. So you must be careful: you don't want to mollycoddle the baby; you don't want to treat every whimper like a national emergency. If you freak out every time your baby so much as gurgles, it'll end up being one of those bratty kids whom you see at hamburger restaurants squealing, "I want fries! I want a party hat! I hate pickles! I want one of those plastic cartoon-character figurines!" But, on the other hand, you don't want to be one of those negligent parents featured on the seven o'clock news because they let their baby scream for two days running.

The great fun that lies ahead for you is the guessing game that you will get to play trying to work out what is "wrong" with your child. You cannot win this game. You see, some babies cry just because they damn well feel like it. And sometimes there is nothing you can do about it.

And then, of course, there is the arch-nemesis of parents everywhere: COLIC.

Colic is one of those things that occur even though no one can explain why, like yawns, sudden pen leaks and reality-television shows.

Colic is a pattern of unstoppable and inexplicable screaming for a few hours every day (usually in the early evening), a few days a week, week after week. These sessions can wear even the most stable and steadfast parents down pretty quickly. When this behaviour starts, it's best to consult your doctor, to confirm that the crying isn't caused by something more serious. Apart from that, you just have to do your best to cope with the noise. See if it's feed-time, check the baby's temperature, cuddle it, talk to it or change its diaper. Counterintuitively, it might be overtired. Babies don't know that, if they're tired, they should just go to sleep. Try seeing if you can settle it down. You can make it more comfortable by massaging it, shoving a binky in its mouth or rocking its cradle. If that doesn't work, get a blanket and go sit in the yard, or take the baby for a walk in the stroller. The screaming never sounds as bad outside the claustrophobic confines of your living room. Why not go to a busy shopping center? It won't necessarily quiet the baby down, but at least you can make others suffer along with you.

If all else fails, you can always sing. When singing, avoid red-blooded renditions of "Here we go, here we go, here we go!" and "It's a Long Way to the Top (If You Wanna Rock 'n' Roll)." Make it gentle, soft and soothing. If you don't know any tunes, make one up — your baby won't know the difference. In fact, you can sing any song you know, as long as you sing it slowly, softly and melodically. Sway back and forth in time to your song and tap a 4/4 beat on the baby's bottom.

This whole crying game needs a lot of patience. A sense of humor doesn't go astray, either. The problem for us guys, as my mother constantly reminds me, is that:

Patience is a virtue, bless it if you can
Always in a woman, never in a man.

Yeah, great. Thanks, Mom. What can I say? Good luck. One day, when your baby is seventeen and asking you for driving lessons and contraceptives, you'll look back on these times as "the easy years."

Of course, most of us can cope with crying babies when it's a sunny day and the birds are singing and we are feeling alert and strong.

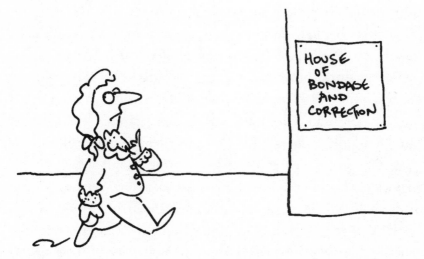

The real test comes at night when you want to sleep.

For many years, political dictators and dungeon-masters have been developing and refining their methods of torture. They have used hot pokers, thumbscrews, the rack, Brahms' *Lullaby* and screenings of *The Fast and the Furious* to make their victims beg for mercy. But there's one form of torture that is used more widely and more effectively than all the others.

Sleep deprivation.

Deprive a man of sleep and he will undergo a Jekyll and Hyde transformation of epic proportions. A normally placid and pleasant Mr. Average can quickly turn into a tired and cranky animal – a short-tempered, bleary-eyed, babbling fool, a rabid and irrational beast. All of a sudden, his whole life is a mess. Unshaven and unkempt, he'll be aggressive to work-mates and fall asleep on the job. He can no longer construct a fluent sentence. His eyelids feel like they are made of lead.

The problem is that babies don't live by the clock or the sun. They don't have the same culturally entrenched ideas about keeping "polite hours." The immediate consequence of this is that they wake up a lot during the night and need to be tended to: fed, burped, changed, rocked to sleep. It's also likely that there'll be a good deal of screaming thrown in for good measure. And when a baby gets a good howl happening in the quiet of the night, it's like a 747 in your bedroom.

I'm not just talking about waking up once for a few minutes in the middle of the night. I know of a couple who called their son The Screamer. He only slept for four hours a day! Gasp! Shock! Snooze! I hear you cry. *Four hours*, did you say? That's inhuman! You're right. It is inhuman. But that's not the worst part. You see, he didn't sleep four hours in one go. That was merely his *cumulative* total. The four hours were made up of occasional twenty-minute snoozes. Meditate on this and you start to realize the impact a baby can have on your household.

Of course, I'm painting a bit of a pessimistic picture. Your baby could alternatively be a marathon sleeper, sleeping as many as eighteen hours in twenty-four. Its cry might only be a barely audible whimper. You may have what is commonly referred to in parenting circles as "a really good baby." If you do, count yourself lucky.

My guess is that, historically, dad went to bed at the normal time and any nocturnal activity of the "waking up and walking around with the baby in the freezing cold dead of night" variety fell under mom's job description. But you need to remember that you are into shared parenting; active fathering. If your wife is at home, she is working all day too and probably never gets a break from the baby and has to put up with that screaming all the time. It is understandable, therefore, that when you walk in the door after "your busy day" and are thinking about putting your feet up, you might be handed a baby by a woman who needs ten minutes to herself.

So, how can *you* help when the baby starts choir practice at 2 am?

When Rachael was born, I thought I had a pretty fool-proof escape clause from any nocturnal activity. My logic was that since I was lacking in the necessary equipment – i.e., one pair of milk-swollen breasts – I was of no use whatsoever and could therefore just roll over and go back to sleep. Of course, I watched my wife gradually turn into a zombie with dark eyes and a blank expression, only capable of monosyllabic conversation. This "It's not my problem" approach is definitely a bad one. (But in my defense, I *did* try to help. Whenever Meredith was up feeding, I would roll over and keep her side of the bed warm.)

When Georgia was born, I vowed to go 50/50. Whenever she got up, I too got up to put on the heater, make hot chocolate and keep her company. This had two immediate effects. First, my presence and talking prevented Georgia from nodding off, which kept us up much longer than necessary. Second, we *both* ended up as zombies with dark eyes and blank expressions, capable only of monosyllabic conversation. And it really is embarrassing to fall asleep at your desk in front of a sophomore class and then wake up to find yourself drooling on your copy of *To Kill a Mockingbird*.

So this "Let's share the torment together" approach is equally inadequate.

So what's the answer?

Without being trite, the answer lies in a balance between the two approaches. It's no good one person doing all the work, but it's no good both of you doing all the work either. Like I said before, parenting is a team game, so share the responsibilities as much as you can. If your baby is being breastfed, play the delivery boy and bring it from the crib to mom in bed. Take turns in burping the baby and singing it off to sleep. This approach worked quite well when we had Matilda. Meredith still did all the feeding, but I tried to help with the burping, settling and pacifier patrol. And when it's not your turn, the best thing you can do is sleep.

To be honest, I rarely lived up to the grandiose expectations I frequently set for myself in the harsh light of day. If you are in a situation where you are going 50/50 with your wife, well, you're a better man than I am, Mr. Din. I think, for most of us, the fact is that our wives still draw the short straw.

Discussion and job-sharing really are the keys to coping. When your wife is fed up, send her out to a movie or for a walk or to a friend's place. And if you're fed up, be sensible enough to accept a break. In BC times (Before Children), whenever I had a spare moment I would fill it with guitar playing or book reading or weight training. In AD times (After Delivery), with a baby in the house, my favorite activity quickly became napping.

But of course it's fine for me to talk about "discussion" and "job-sharing" as if they're the answer to all your night-time troubles. The reality of getting up to a crying baby may be somewhat different. And it's only at this point that I warn you about something . . .

Puttering around with a baby, especially in the middle of the night, can be really frustrating. The crying is harder to cope with because all is quiet, and this only exacerbates the shrill pitch of the baby's cry. It's dark and still and you feel like you're the only person on Earth who's awake. You feel even more lonely and isolated because often the only company you have in the wee hours are the people in infomercials for home-gym equipment, low-fat barbecue hotplates and inde-structible sunglasses. And that's enough to drive anybody crazy.

Of course, we all start out well enough, but it doesn't take long before you can start to feel out of sorts and then lose your temper. I had read about this in books, but because I am a mature, highly-educated and well-adjusted guy – a parenting author, even! – I knew that this would not be a problem for me.

But it was. This dawned on me in the early hours one morning as I was playing a lengthy game called "putting Georgia back to bed after a midnight feed." Every night, Meredith and I played this game. That night, it was my turn. I stood there next to her crib, trying to sway her off to sleep. (Georgia, that is, not Meredith.) It was cold. It was dark. It was quiet. Pretty soon, I was fighting to keep my eyes open and ended up slumped against the wall, my face pressed into the wallpaper, and mumbling some inane lullaby.

Eventually, after what seemed like hours but was probably only minutes, she dozed off. I then had to endure the perilous and nerve-wracking challenge of trying to lower her into the crib and get my arm out without waking her – an activity best illustrated in action movies when some sweaty and trem-bling government agent has to carefully remove some sort of incredibly sensitive beeping electronic thing from a metal housing in a bomb and if he so much as breathes too heavily then his arm will jolt and a warning light will start flashing and ten seconds later there'll be a nuclear explosion. Mission accomplished, I spent several minutes backing out down the corridor to my bedroom, like a kung-fu master on rice paper. I made it to within a few tantalizing feet of the warmth of my bed before I hit that creaky floorboard. Then she cranked up again. A piercing howl in the darkness.

She had just been fed, so she wasn't hungry.

She had just been changed, so she wasn't wet.

She was wrapped in a blanket, so she wasn't cold.

So I went back and started gently rocking the crib. I mean, I was doing it by the book. But she was still screaming as if I were taunting her with red-hot irons. I started singing. And rocking. Singing and rocking.

This had worked well before, but on this occasion . . . it didn't.

Singing and rocking.

It was dark and I was tired and her scream was like fingernails on a chalkboard. I started getting angry. My best attempts at baby-soothing had been frustrated. Her scream was deafening. My feet were cold. My eyes were sore. So I rocked harder. It still didn't work.

Suddenly, I felt a volcano of frustration welling up inside me. I wanted to bang the crib hard and make the crying stop and run outside and rip up trees by their trunks and smash armoured vehicles with my fists, just like the Incredible Hulk. I was losing control. Somewhere in the back of my brain, an alarm bell started ringing. So I backed outa there and went and splashed some water on my face and took a few deep breaths. Then I took Georgia into the lounge room, put the TV and the heater on and started the singing/rocking routine again. Being in a warm, bright room made me wake up a bit and feel better, and, more importantly, cope a whole lot better.

You should be aware of this nocturnal frustration. It is real. There are ways of coping, however. Put on some calming music and make some toast. Put on headphones and walk your baby around the house. I know a couple who used to put their baby in its car seat and go for a drive. The noise and rhythm of the car soothed the baby and sent it off to sleep. (Just make sure *you* don't fall asleep at the wheel.) Another couple I know get up, put their baby in a sling and vacuum the house. The noise drowns out the screams, the house gets clean and the baby is eventually soothed by the rhythm. What more could you ask for?

If you start "losing it," put the baby in its crib where it can't hurt itself and go back to bed, or get in the shower or even open your back door and go outside and take ten deep breaths or do some chin-ups or whatever it takes to shake you out of the funk. If things are really bad, don't be afraid or embarrassed to phone up a compliant friend or relative to come and help you out. There are various telephone helplines in each state that can offer support and advice. Look them up online and stick their phone numbers to the side of your fridge.

Of course, it all depends on whether your baby is a dozer or a screamer and how well you and your wife handle sleep deprivation. But have the attitude of helping. Take it in turns to deal with the baby, and discuss what suits your situation best. And work out in advance some coping strategies for if it ever seems too much.

And, good luck, my friend. You'll need it.

SIDS

SIDS stands for sudden infant death syndrome.

The definition of SIDS on the sidsandkids.org website is:

> The sudden and unexpected death of an infant under one year of age, with onset of the fatal episode apparently occurring during sleep, that remains unexplained after a thorough investigation including performance of a complete autopsy, and review of the circumstances of death and the clinical history.

What this means in layman's terms is that some babies die in their sleep and no one knows why.

SIDS is the most common form of death for babies between one month and one year of age, with the ages of one to six months accounting for over eighty percent of these. However, a combination of intensive medical research and large-scale public-awareness campaigns has meant that, since 1994, when Healthy Child Care America introduced the "Back to Sleep" campaign, the number of deaths has dropped massively. While still a tragic figure, the current rate of SIDS in the United States has dropped to about 2,000 per year.

While no one knows what causes SIDS, research has provided us with practices that will reduce the chance of its occurring. These are good for you to know, and it is certainly worth your while doing some more extensive reading on this subject. Brochures are readily available from hospitals and birth classes, and there are many websites (including sids.org) that provide specific details and advice.

So what can you do to reduce the chance of your baby dying of SIDS? In the first place, babies should sleep on their backs in a crib that is free of junk. There should be no electric blankets, water bottles, pillows, stuffed toys, bumpers, quilts, blankets, ribbons or any other loose bedding or toys in there. Ensure the mattress is firm and well fitted. A baby should be tucked in securely, with its face clearly uncovered. A fitted baby sleeping bag is ideal. The baby's feet should be at the base of the crib so that it has little chance of burrowing down under the covers. This gives the impression of a huge empty space at the head of the bed, but that's fine.

Smoking is also a highly influential factor, with babies of smokers significantly more likely to die of SIDS than babies of non-smokers. So if you're a smoker, there's no time like now to give up.

If you are having a babysitter look after your baby, make sure that they are clear on the above information. Things may well have been different in Grandma's day and she is probably not as up to speed as you are on current SIDS advice. ("Listen, my boy, I used to pop you face down and bury you in your crib with your favorite blanket and all your teddy bears, and you turned out all right!")

Splish Splash

Babies have to be washed. If you don't wash them, they'll start to smell and not be so much fun to have around.

A quick and easy option is the frequently used "top 'n' tail," where the baby's face and bum get a nice once over with a cloth. But if you use the same cloth for both bits, make sure you wash the baby's face first.

Every so often, though, your baby is going to need a proper bath. You can do this in a "safe" sink (i.e. free of taps sticking out at skull-cracking angles and with no danger of hot taps coming on), or in a baby bath (as mentioned in Chapter Four), placed on a sturdy bench or table or on the floor. If you're game, and if you have one, you can take the baby in the big bath with you. However, you have to do some prep and be careful getting in and out, and ensure the temperature is okay.

You must be very careful with the water temperature. If you have the baby in the bath with you, the temperature must be set for the baby, not for you. What *you* consider a normal, nice, relaxing bath after your hard day at work could be lethal to your baby, because they don't have the same temperature tolerance as you. This applies to both hot and cold baths. (Like in the same way your favorite chili feast or icy drink would burn your baby's throat.)

A bath a baby is getting into should be pleasantly and mildly warm, not hot. But how do you get the temperature right? The traditional method is to test the water with your wrist or elbow, because your hands are apparently too weathered. (I've wondered, about this, though, because my elbow is as tough as elephant hide and has the sensitivity of concrete. But generations of parents swear by it.) There is, of course, one part of your body that we both know is very sensitive to extreme water-temperature immersion, but it's not very practical just to get it out and dangle it in. Some friends of mine use a baby-bath thermometer that floats in the bath and turns different colors if the water is too hot or too cold. Probably overkill, but they like it.

Okay, here comes the big thing to remember. If this is the only thing you get out of this book, so be it. Here it is in bold, italics and underlined for triple emphasis: ***Never leave your baby alone in the bath, not even for a second.***

Every year, babies drown because mom or dad quickly went to answer the phone or turn off the stove or even just turned around to get a towel. Babies can drown in just a few centimeters of water, and all it takes is the time for them to draw one single breath. So, once again, ***never leave your baby alone in the bath, not even for a second.*** Put your phone on silent. Turn off the stove first. Ignore the knock at the door. Keep the water shallow. You also need to take care to support your baby's lolling head in the early months, ensuring its mouth is above the water at all times.

Set up the bath and dressing area with everything you need *before* you bring the baby into the picture. That way, you won't be tempted to leave your baby alone in the water or on the changing table while you go hunting for this or that.

When dressing a baby after its bath, get the diaper on first, particularly if your baby is a boy. Boys have a defense system that transforms their penis into a high-pressure directional urine squirter that has its own locking mechanism and is constantly aimed at your face. (You'd be surprised how many guys have emailed me to say, "I thought you were kidding!" I'm not.) Forewarned is forearmed (with a diaper).

Twenty-One Days of Diapers

To many men, fatherhood is a scary prospect. They are nervous about all the awesome changes and responsibilities that accompany family life. There are also new financial pressures, a major change to the daily timetable, lack of sleep and more household chores. But to most men there is one thing that is scarier than all these other concerns put together. It is worse than any horror film; the stuff of which nightmares are made.

It is . . . diapers. Mountains of festering, smoldering ones.

Your baby is going to go through about 6000 diapers, which, at five minutes a change, means you'll be cumulatively elbow deep for about 500 hours, or twenty-one whole days of your life.

Diapers are incredible. Like an ant with a distended abdomen in a David Attenborough documentary, babies can carry around in their diapers over a hundred times their own body weight. This is frightening, because then they need to be changed.

I still remember the first time I saw a friend change his baby's diaper. I was a "diaper virgin" and, when he opened that bad boy up, I immediately went into "diaper shock," also known in psych texts as PDTS, or "post-diaper traumatic syndrome." I sat on my friend's front steps, sweaty-faced and hyperventilating. He laughed at me and said, "It's okay, mate. I used to be like that. It's always bad with somebody else's kid. But your own kids – you get used to it."

Tom Selleck, in the classic film *Three Men and a Baby*, sums up the sentiment nicely: when faced with the prospect of changing another diaper, he offers his mate Steve Guttenberg a thousand dollars to do it for him. Some might argue this is a good value for the money.

It's no use thinking that you can make it through the early years of your baby's life without changing one. You can't. (I tried, but Meredith soon became suspicious that every time a diaper needed changing, I was suddenly asleep, in the bathroom or hiding under the kitchen table.) As an involved twenty-first-century dad experiencing fatherhood in all its glory, you have to "get your hands dirty" (metaphorically and literally). Being a dad is more than doing all the fun jobs like kicking a ball in the backyard and sharing your paternal wisdom around a campfire. Diaper changing, despite the opinion of many, is not an innately maternal pastime.

My first diaper changes were memorable.

I have a steel stomach, current First Aid certification and have seen every Sylvester Stallone film ever made. But I went to jelly in the face of my first diapers. In fact, I dry-retched. I didn't realize it at the time, but these were to be the first in a long line of reverse-peristalsis experiences in the presence of Diapers from Hell.

Over its first few days, the baby's waste is a disgusting, greeny-black, sticky, festering mess called meconium. You'll look at it and think, "How did this massive glob of congealed engine oil get into that diaper?" This is the crap version of the amniotic fluid and bile and other goop that the baby has ingested in the womb. Don't let it come into contact with your skin, carpet, clothing or small pets. Seriously. That stuff does not come off.

Once the baby's system is cleaned out and the breastmilk has worked its way through, the diapers improve markedly, relatively speaking. For the first few months, the baby will produce a seemingly impossible volume of wet, sloppy, gooey fluid, the kind you'd expect as the result of having a purely liquid diet. (If meconium is tar, then milk-fed poo is gravy.)

But down the track, once the baby starts eating solids (especially meat), then you're in real trouble. That's when you have to deal with fair-dinkum solid crap, perfectly molded into rhomboidal patties in the airspace formed by the baby's buttocks and diaper. These craps have their own label in the periodic table of elements: 113 Excretium (Ex), with an atomic weight of 272.03.

It turns out that my friend was right, and, although difficult at first, you do get used to it. A veteran of three babies, by Tilly's last diaper (a champagne moment, by the way), I could change the most nuclear diaper with my bare hands – in the dark, even, although that's not recommended. I've even seen parent veterans just drive their finger deep down the back of a diaper to check if it needs changing.

When cleaning your baby's bum, use disposable, moist towelettes or cotton balls and water to wipe away the slimy poop that is smeared on its skin. Some bits might need some elbow grease, because, if you've left it too long, little poopy flecks will have dried out and set like concrete. Also, make sure you gently get down inside the folds of loose skin around the bum and thighs. If the bum is red and rashy, you can apply some barrier cream or baby cream to help soothe and protect the irritated skin.

Apart from that, when changing diapers there are two rules:

Rule One: Securely Fasten the New Diaper

A loose diaper can drop off of its own accord. Older babies can also work out how to take them off. Use electrical tape, an arc welder, superglue – whatever it takes to make the diaper secure. If you don't, your baby will use the chunky stuff as paint or modelling clay . . . or worse. Trust me, it's not easy bonding with a baby who has crap around its mouth.

Rule Two: Hold Your Breath

The current world record for holding one's breath (without pure-oxygen supercharging) is over eleven minutes. That is more than enough time to change a diaper. Start building up your lung capacity now. If you happen to suck in a lungful of contaminated diaper air without breathing apparatus, drink milk and seek medical advice.

Diaper Types

When trying to work out what sort of diapers you might use on your baby, there are a number of factors to consider: convenience, comfort, dryness, expense, eco-friendliness and what all your friends are doing. It really does boil down to personal preference, with the internet rife with parents flying the flag one way or another and declaring that *this* type of diaper is cheaper, better for the environment and drier, while others claim the exact opposite. Experiment a bit yourself.

In your role as diaper changer, you have four options.

Option 1: Cloth Diapers

Things sure have come a long way in the cloth-diaper market. When Rachael was first born, cloth diapers were giant, terry-towelling squares that, after an elaborate origami-esque folding procedure, were wrapped fatly around the baby, causing a ridiculously bulbous bow-legged effect. Not only that, prior to the invention of the three-pronged "snappy," they were secured in place with big safety pins. This was a nightmare, particularly when the pin burst through the cloth and speared deep under your fingernail. ("Infection? Let *me* tell *you* about infection!")

Modern cloth diapers are now "fitted" and therefore faster and easier to put on. Fans of cloth like the feel and smell of the cotton and consider it more natural and eco-friendly than disposables. They are also easier to clean. Back in the day, you had to scrape the excra-pattie off the cloth, which generally had formed a frustrating covalent bond with the fabric. Now, you can use a biodegradable bamboo liner to roll up the bad stuff and send it down the toilet.

Initially, you need to buy a couple of large buckets with lids and a tower of diapers. After a soiled diaper is emptied, throw it in the bucket for a soak in sterilizing fluid. (As these are germ killers, they are not particularly good for the environment, so if you are on your own septic system, avoid emptying the bucket into it.) After an overnight soak, throw the diapers in your washing machine with a good detergent. Hanging the diapers out in the sun will bleach even the most lurid yellow ones white. It sounds complex and time-consuming, but once you have a regular system up and running, it's really quite simple.

On top of that, if cloth is your preference but you don't want to muck about with all the washing, try a diaper service.

They provide all the gear (bucket, diapers, liners, inserts, etc.) and then once or twice a week will arrive at your door to drop off a giant bag of fresh, clean diapers. At the same time, they'll take away a giant bag of sodden, sludgy ones. (Of course, this gets more fun as the week goes on and the bag fills up – particularly in summer. This is also a great way of getting back at neighbors you don't like who live downwind from you. Even better, it keeps door-to-door salesmen and various religious cults away.)

If you have a friend or relative who wants to buy you a present but isn't sure what to get you, a couple of weeks' worth of diaper service will be a gift you'll really appreciate.

One more thing: some cloth users are fans because they claim disposables are bad for the environment (landfill, etc.) and therefore cloth is a more eco-friendly choice. While there is some merit in this, critics point out that the water, energy and detergents used in cleaning cloth diapers also have a significant, if hidden, environmental impact.

Option 2: Disposable Diapers

We live in a fast-paced convenience-centric culture where so much of our consumerism is *use and throw*: pens, takeout containers, drink bottles, razors, napkins, tea bags, coffee pods, cameras, plates and cutlery, and, of course, diapers.

American parents have taken to disposable diapers like a Mexico tourist to a sombrero. They may cost more than cloth, but they are quick and convenient to use. When they're "soiled," the responsible and hygienic thing to do is to scrape the gunk off into the toilet before discarding the diaper. (That stuff shouldn't go to the dump; it should go to the sewage plant.) Then you simply wrap them up and throw them away.

This is particularly advantageous if you are out for the day and don't wish to carry around a plastic bag of fermenting sludge.

Fans of disposables also describe them as having less impact on the household, as well as being better fitting, which means they are less bulky and have less leakage, and being more absorbent, which keeps the baby drier.

However, some parents don't like the chemical smell and feel of some disposables. And then there's cost. Babies go through diapers about as quickly as you can put them on. At first, your baby will use about seven to ten diapers a day; maybe more, maybe less. This is going to cost you a tidy sum, especially considering that babies are in diapers for about two years. And if your garbage is only collected once a week, you will soon find that the sauna-like effect of the wheelie bin on the seventy or so little packets will lead to a marital dispute as to who gets to put the trash out. And the garbage crew will hate you too.

And in case you think that selecting disposable diapers is easy, think again. There are disposables for newborns, infants, crawlers, toddlers and juniors, diapers for boys, diapers for girls and even "non-ballooning" secure diapers for the swimming pool. There are more varieties of diapers than there are types of dog food – all with computer-designed, color-coded, sex-differentiated, scientifically proven features that will take your baby's bum through the next millennium, oft with impressive and fancy patented names like "Leak Block," "Absorbo-Max," "Tab-Grip," "Wet-Lock System" and "Dry-Guard-Plus."

American babies' diapers contribute several million tons to landfills each year. Critics tell us that disposables have the same half-life as toxic waste. Which is not surprising, considering that diapers *contain* toxic waste. They will still be intact and lethal at the local rubbish dump in a million years when the aliens finally get here, and all that will be left of our civilization will be mounds of diapers. Having said that, the disposability of diapers has improved and there is a range of eco-disposables on the market for the eco-warrior in all of us.

Option 3: The Diaper Combo
No, not a new meal deal from your local hamburger restaurant ("Would you like any desserts with your diaper, sir?"). Some parents use a combination of both disposable and cloth diapers. With this, you get the best of both worlds: cloth diapers during the day and around the house; disposable diapers at night and for trips away from home.

Option 4: No Diaper
We have (shall we say *earthy*) friends who decided not to restrict their baby by having it wear diapers. They wanted it to be free and didn't like the idea of it having to be sitting in a bag of its own waste. Nice in theory, but the short version is that their carpet and soft-furnishings are not what they once were and we try not to visit them anymore.

Option 4 is not recommended.

No matter what option you choose, however, invest in a diaper-changing outfit. A wetsuit, oxygen tank, welding mask, blacksmith's gloves and a wooden spoon will do you nicely. Or, if you have a spare room, build one of those uranium-shielded handling rooms where you can change your baby using robotic arms from behind the safety of a glass panel.

8

Living with a Baby

"It's not that your life comes to a complete standstill.
It's more a shifting down through the gears
without using a clutch."

Do Not Feed the Animal

Once you have navigated your way through the earliest days of keeping your baby healthy, happy and alive, you will find it has developed sufficiently to present you with a whole new raft of things to consider. One such development/concern is teething. If you stick your finger in your baby's mouth any time in the first six months, you will notice that it feels more like a fish than a tiger. There are no teeth. But it doesn't stay like that forever. Around the half-year mark, the first of twenty little white splinters will drive their way through your baby's gums. This is its first set of teeth, which it will have for about six years.

This has many immediate effects:

- Your baby will drool. There will be a continuous river of saliva running from its lower lip down to its navel, giving your baby a glistening appearance.
- Your baby may be very uncomfortable. It may be whiny and miserable and have difficulty settling or sleeping sometimes.
- If your wife breastfeeds, you will hear her yelp intermittently as the baby's carnivorous instincts impact upon her nipples.
- The baby will produce diapers of such suffocating intensity and revolting consistency that you will redefine your understanding of nausea.
- When (not if) your baby bites you, it will hurt.

Now, this is all part of the natural order, because a newborn baby only drinks milk so doesn't need teeth. But over the course of its first year, your baby will start its journey towards real food. This process is called weaning, whereby its milk intake is lowered and solids are gradually phased in. (I use the term "solids" very loosely. To me, a solid is a rump steak with fries. To baby-food manufacturers, however, a solid is a banana that has spent an hour in a blender.)

A baby should be breastfed (or bottle fed) exclusively for its first six months, before weaning begins. But don't expect it to take place overnight. It is a slow process. Be guided by your baby. If it shows interest in foods, or if it isn't gaining in weight as it ought to be, or if it has reached six months of age, start on solids. To begin, only one or two teaspoons of food should be offered once a day for the first couple of weeks, and then you build from there. These early foods should be bland, wet and slushy, such as rice cereal, fruit and vegetable purée and gels.

Don't give too much food at any one sitting – breastmilk should still be its main source of nutrition up to six months and even beyond – and introduce new foods slowly, feeding each new type for two or three days running to check for possible allergic reactions before introducing the next food.

And it's also around this teething time that you can introduce teething biscuits, which are little sticks of flavored concrete that babies use to sharpen their teeth on so when they bite you they get a better response.

With this onset of teeth, your baby can start on foods of a more resilient consistency. You can throw your whole dinner into a blender and give them a semi-solid goulash of homemade baby fare. Later on, you can introduce them to actual pieces of bread, cheese, (boned) fish, chicken, veggies, hamburger, fruits . . . in fact, pretty well anything off your dinner plate will do, as long as it's not beef vindaloo, chili chicken or jalapeno burritos.

One of the problems with introducing solids is that babies like to experiment with their food. This usually involves putting it in their mouth, chewing it, spitting it out, picking it up, rubbing it into their clothes, throwing some of it into your face, running it through their hair before putting it back in their mouth again and blowing bubbles through it. Unfortunately, only a bit of food actually ends up in your baby's stomach. It would be awesome and convenient if babies could simply get the nutrition out of their food via the process of osmosis, whereby the vitamins and minerals soak directly through their skin, but this is not so. But don't give up. This is all part of the slow process of a baby learning what to do with food.

And so, be aware: this can all make a bit of a mess. Feed your baby over linoleum or tiles, or in the center of a plastic tablecloth, and never near a pile of fresh washing/ironing. Even then, you will still find morsels of food splattered inexplicably on the ceiling on the other side of the room.

To protect the baby's clothing, many people use bibs. These are cheap, which means all your friends will buy you ten packs each as a present and you'll need a separate cupboard to store them in. But bibs are peculiar things, inasmuch as they don't work. Babies will get food down their sleeves and in their socks, and no tiny piece of cloth with cute bunny prints is going to stop them. So not only will you need to wash their clothes (which you would have done anyway), you'll also need to wash hundreds of bibs as well, increasing your washing load by 200 percent.

Out and About

With the baby's patterns of feeding, sleeping and soiling diapers, getting out the front door isn't as easy as it used to be. Even simple things like visiting a friend or going to the store suddenly become more complicated. It's not that your life comes to a complete standstill. It's more a shifting down through the gears without using a clutch. But you'll have to start getting out eventually, otherwise you'll run out of food.

In your pre-baby years, going out was relatively simple. In fact, you could probably make it out of the house in seconds. Splash water on your face, find some cash and a clean shirt, grab your car keys and wallet – thirty seconds, tops. It doesn't work like this anymore. Operation Desert Storm was easier to coordinate than Operation Getting Out the Front Door. This is organization on a grand scale.

The baby has to be put in a clean diaper, dressed, bundled up and held. The holder now has only one arm. The bag has to be packed with a blanket, extra diapers, plastic bags, bottles, pacifiers, creams, gels, a change of clothes, stuffed toys with jingly bells, and so on. The car seat has to be refitted and the stroller folded into the trunk. The travel crib needs to be packed down and squashed into whatever available space you have left. (By the way, tech schools offer Engineering diplomas specializing in travel-crib construction.)

Once supply lines have been established, there's the plan of attack to consider. If you're going to your mother-in-law's for lunch, for example, make your estimated time of departure an hour earlier than normal. That way, you'll ensure that you only miss the first course. Because just when you're ready to go, you can bet that your baby will need a feed.

And if it's a really big night – somewhere your baby just can't go – you need to start planning days in advance. A babysitter needs to be organized and, if your wife is breastfeeding, an adequate supply of breastmilk expressed and stored.

Going out with your baby is a great way of spending time together and giving it something new to look at, whether it be a trip to the store, a walk in the park, hanging out with friends, grabbing a coffee, or just going around the block to get some fresh air. There's one other thing that you must remember, though. A newborn's skin is about one thousand times more sensitive than your leathery hide. This is not helped by the depletion of the ozone layer. A baby can burn easily, even on a cloudy day. I am still surprised at how often I see parents (wearing shades and hats) walking or jogging along, oblivious to the fact that their baby in the stroller in front of them is being blasted by full midday sunlight.

And I shouldn't need to say this but, for the sake of being thorough, never put your baby out to sunbathe. (In fact, never put *anyone* out to sunbathe.) This particularly applies to visits to the pool or beach. Avoid exposure to the sun, especially in the middle of the day, and always ensure your baby is wearing a sunscreen with a sun-protection factor (SPF) of 30+, plus a hat and sun shirt. Also, put a hand towel or shade-screen in your car window to stop the sun frying your baby in its car seat. Make sure, though, that you put the towel on a *side* window, not the *front* window. This will improve your driving visibility significantly.

Let's Party

Babies are a lot of work. It's important, however, that you don't get so absorbed by the maintenance duties and chores that you forget to actually *enjoy* them. Have some fun and play with your infant so the two of you can get to know each other and build a relationship. (Although it's hard to think ahead now, this is laying critical foundations and patterns that will bring big rewards in later years.)

"Play" does not mean shoving lots of expensive toys in its face or finding the latest baby-activity app. Know this: your child's best ever toy is . . . you.

Don't wait till it can catch a ball. Play starts immediately and should be pitched at the baby's level, not yours (i.e., lots of contact but no contact sports). Be inventive, laugh a lot, don't do anything that will frighten it and, without wanting to bust out the scented candles, simply be in the moment with them, just hanging out together. Oh, and keep one hand over your testicles at all times.

Play for Newborn Babies
- Having a massage.
- Being held.
- Looking at your face.
- Being talked to.
- Being sung to.
- Swaying.
- Watching you jostle stuffed toys with jingly bells while you make non-threatening silly faces.

Play for Older Babies
- Chewing (teething rings, bananas, phones).
- Making faces.
- Making silly noises.
- Rolling around on the floor or bed.
- Cuddles.
- Drooling on dad.
- Urinating on dad.
- Vomiting on dad.
- Knee bounces.
- Clapping and singing songs.
- Peek-a-boo.
- Getting raspberries on the stomach.
- Being tickled.
- Squeaky toys and picture books.
- Going for trips in the stroller or backpack.

- Gentle throwing up in the air. (Beware ceiling fans).
- And again, massage.

Spend time with your baby from Day One. Engage in physical contact. Cuddle your baby, hold its hands and stroke its hair. Touch and massage are very important factors in helping your baby to thrive and feel loved. Find a quiet, warm place and use some baby oil to gently massage your baby's arms and legs, hands and feet, back and stomach. Let it fall asleep on your chest. Skin to skin contact is a really important way of connecting with your baby. Let it get used to (in the words of Champ Kind) "your musk."

Sing to your baby. Talk to it. Let it hear your voice. But, whatever you do, don't converse in what you think is its own language. I do not understand why adults persist in doing this. I mean, how would you feel if the only way people communicated with you was in a musical voice chiming, "Bootchie-wootchie-coo-coo. Bubba wanna car-car? Daddy lo-o-o-o-o-o-ves his baby bitsy poo-poo. YeeeEEEsssss? Ah gubbagubbagubbagubba . . ."

If your baby starts crying, it's 'cause they just realized their dad is an idiot.

I always just talked to my kids as if they knew what I was talking about, especially when complaining about work (#captiveaudience).

Also, having something of a penchant for music myself, I always enjoyed singing nursery rhymes to my children. But be warned. Many nursery rhymes were composed by people with some serious issues, often back in the Dark Ages, when the major food staples were bone marrow, moss, hair and boiled shoe leather.

Case in point: "Rock-a-Bye-Baby," a child-abuse song about a baby who has been put in its cradle – not in a nice, warm bedroom but in a *treetop*. Despite the fact the author knows that "when the wind blows, the cradle will rock," up into the tree the baby goes. Predictably, the branch breaks during a storm, and the baby and cradle crash through the canopy in an arboreal heap, probably with significant injuries.

In fact, most nursery rhymes have some oddball origin in the past. "Ring a Ring a Rosy" is a ditty about kids with necrotic flesh dying during the bubonic plague. They start sneezing ("atishoo, atishoo"), which spreads their germs and they "all fall down," as in dead. And then there's the one about the dude who puts twenty-four *live* blackbirds in a pie and bakes them, so that when the King cuts open the pie, the birds all start singing. Seriously, imagine cutting into a pie and finding those birds all balled up with their sweaty feathers and desperate, boggly eyes, entombed in a pastry inferno. That is seriously messed up. Don't even get me started with Miss Muffet, who was minding her own business, sitting on a grassy knob, snacking on some cottage cheese, when a giant freaking spider turned up next to her.

Then again, at least they have a narrative, unlike some other traditional offerings. I once found myself reading the following to my children:

Pussy cat ate the dumplings,
Shu-o-a, shu-o-a, oh fie.
Poussie, poussie boudrons.
I got a wee mousie
And put it in my meal-poke
And nar shan't gar me gang down
Shu-o-a, shu-o-a, oh fie.

It's amazing that my kids turned out okay in the end.

An alternative is to make up your own songs. I always use established tunes but free-associate my own words. Remember, it doesn't really matter *what* you sing; it's the *way* you sing it that matters. For example, to the tune of "Old MacDonald Had a Farm':

The pasta on the stove is ready,
Ee-eye, ee-eye, oh.
I want to check the baseball score,
Ee-eye, ee-eye, oh.
There's a fly in the room,
I'm gonna squash it flat,
Then I'm going for a walk
and I really hate this wallpaper.
Hurry up and go to sleep,
Ee-eye, ee-eye, oh.

Or to the tune of "Amazing Grace':

I'm wearing jeans and you are not,
My tax is due today,
The weather is nice,
My phone won't synch,
And my favorite TV show is Survivor.

Hey, you can't blame a guy for trying.

Hurry Up and Wait!

When Rachael came home from the hospital, I was keen to be the happy dad, just like in the glossy mags and movies; Cuddles, wrestles on the carpet, throwing my daughter in the air, lots of laughter, fun and tummy-tickling, making faces, walks in the park (for some reason in movies, always in slo-mo with a funky soundtrack), and eventually crying at her university graduation when she threw her mortarboard in the air. This was all well and good, but it didn't take me long to discover that newborn babies are . . . well . . . sedate.

Some would even say boring.

Newborn babies don't do much. They have four basic functions, which they repeat with monotonous regularity. They:

1. Sleep (somewhere around sixteen hours a day, if you are blessed).
2. Cry (a lot, when they're not drinking milk or asleep).
3. Drink milk (when they're not crying or asleep).
4. Excrete (pretty well constantly).

At first, I was slightly miffed that my backyard camp-outs, fatherly lectures and chainsaw lessons would have to wait until Rachael was more mature. But then, in the depth of my despair, something wonderful happened. I'm not doting or sentimental, but, one day, some time after the homecoming, Rachael wrapped her minute hand around my index finger and squeezed it like she was milking a cow.

That single little action was a ray of light that made me realize I was privy to the growth of a little person. At that stage, she really did nothing except the usual sleep, cry, drink and crap routine, but I suddenly realized that in the coming months I would see her grow, change and develop. I would see her come to recognize me. I would watch her first steps. I would hear her first words. I was important. I was her dad.

And that is exactly what happened. Three times now.

Like I said, I'm not doting or sentimental and had no previous interest in babies, but when it comes to your own, somehow, mystically, the rules change. Turns out it is quite thrilling to participate in the life and growth of a baby. Who'd have thought?

Problem is, our consumer world has sold us into a culture of impatience. I want everything *now*. Be it a takeout coffee, movies on demand, the big corner office or fruit out of season, we have lost some of our ability *to wait*.

When it comes to your own child's development, don't expect everything at once. I must admit that I spent a bit of time staring at each of my kids, camera poised, waiting for their next important developmental milestone to occur. And as soon as the baby even moved, I'd start recording. And I'm sure I'm not the first dad who, when their one-year-old beat the keys of a piano with clenched fists, yelled out, "Did you hear that? Did you hear that? Beethoven's *Fifth*! Child prodigy!"

One day, Rachael was lying on her stomach during her third month. Her leg went into a spasm and kicked out – the way babies' legs do – and she nudged forward an inch. The next day, I told a colleague at work that Rachael was starting to crawl even though she was only two months old. She looked at me with the tolerant and knowing smile of parental experience. Her face said it all: "Over-excited new dad with ridiculously high expectations."

Growing up is a slow and laborious process. Your baby won't do everything overnight. But, that's part of the fun.

So what exactly can you expect, and when? Well, here's a rough guide to the developmental stages of babies. Remember, though, that I'm not a medical doctor or a child psychologist or anything like that. The following list is less the result of any serious empirical analysis and more the result of watching babies down at the local playgroup.

At zero months, you can expect your baby to:

- cry, drink, vomit, crap, sleep (repeat)
- lie on the carpet, rug or bed
- get gifts of stuffed toys and bibs from your friends.

At three months, you can expect your baby to:

- smile
- shake a rattle
- play with its hands
- start to lift its head
- be responsive to you.

At six months, you can expect your baby to:

- start getting teeth
- bite you with its teeth (see previous)
- produce "teething diapers" (oh, the horror, the horror)
- use hands to pick up disgusting objects
- use hands to put disgusting objects into mouth
- eat foods other than breastmilk
- gurgle and sing to itself
- sit up for a few seconds without bashing its head on the floor
- use an iPad for the first time.

At nine months, you can expect your baby to:

- sit up
- stand up by holding onto things
- crawl
- never shut up
- amaze your dinner-party friends with its ability to work iPad apps, generally involving cartoon animals, annoying sounds and colorful shapes.

At twelve months, you can expect your baby to:

- recognize its name
- eat finger food
- remove its own diaper and eat anything it finds within
- walk with the assistance of a walker trolley
- stumble from walker trolley and smack head into wall
- bite you a lot
- throw tantrums in public places.

At fifteen months, you can expect your baby to:

- use basic words
- stumble dangerously around at high speeds
- eat small, cut-up bits of what you eat
- have favorite toys or books
- get into places where it shouldn't be
- nod to indicate *yes* and *no*, and wave goodbye
- own shoes that are more expensive than yours.

At eighteen months, you can expect your baby to:

- point at things it wants
- demand to have your attention all the time
- understand basic commands, such as "No!" and "Fetch!"
- break or flush something very valuable (phone)
- contract a mystery illness that will make you very worried
- take half an hour to get it dressed, thanks to its non-cooperation.

At twenty-four months, you can expect your baby to:

- start to use a "big" toilet, with some assistance
- use a spoon
- play by itself
- have a basic vocabulary and primitive sentence construction
- have a junk-food addiction
- use a mouse.

At thirty months, you can expect your baby to:

- ask you perplexing questions such as:
  - Where is the world?
  - Why is red?
  - Am I a tree?
  - What happened before this day?
- ride a pedal tricycle
- know the jingle from every irritating commercial on TV.

At thirty-six months, you can expect your baby to:

- read a couple of words
- stumble into your bedroom every night
- operate complicated home-entertainment-unit remote controls
- know what foods it dislikes
- show you how to change the settings on your laptop or smartphone
- strike up conversations with strangers at the supermarket, generally kicking off with:
  - You're fat!
  - Where's your hair?
  - Are you chocolate?
  - Do you have a penis? My dad does.
  - Why is your skin so wrinkly?

At 108 months, you can expect your baby to:

- ask for pocket money
- want a horse or drum kit for Christmas
- want every stuffed animal at the county fair
- come out with its first swear words.

At 144 months, you can expect your baby to:

- want to get its ears pierced
- get a phone call from school saying they posted an inappropriate comment on a social media website about one of their friends, who is now quite upset
- run faster than you.

At 180 months, you can expect your baby to:

- bring home its first love, whom you won't like
- want to get its navel/eyebrow/nose pierced
- spend hours in the bathroom dicking about with product or a straightener.

At 192 months, you can expect your baby to:

- get its driver's license.

At 216 months, you can expect your baby to:

- see an R-rated film
- come home at 2 am and get grounded for ten years
- want to borrow your car.

At 252 months, you can expect your baby to:

- drink alcohol legally
- be earning more than you
- have a baby of their own.

Yep, as they get older, it just gets better. This way, like a fine wine, you enjoy it more.

By the way, your child will never perform any of their new feats in front of guests. Your baby may be able to clap hands or play peek-a-boo. It might be able to stand on its head, discuss environmental issues in a second language, sing opera or perform complex mathematical functions while tap-dancing. But the moment guests arrive at your place, it will not cooperate. You will ask it to do things and it will stare at you dumbly, and your friends will raise their eyebrows at you.

So when you have guests over, never say, "Baby David . . . come here . . . yes, yes . . . come on, that's the boy! Tell Aunty Sue the square root of nine."

Your baby will look at you and invariably respond with, "DOG!"

Aunty Sue shuffles awkwardly.

"C'mon, you know the answer . . . *please*," you beg.

"SNOT!"

"Well, um . . . thanks for a great night," says Aunty Sue.

And be assured that the moment Sue steps out the door, your baby will look you in the eye and say, "Three."

Secure the House

Once things have settled down a bit in your home and the two of you are getting used to being the three of you, there are some further changes you'll need to make around the place.

As I mentioned earlier, newborns don't move around much by themselves. With the exception of changing tables, they basically lie wherever you leave them, like a turtle on its back. Therefore, they don't really have much of an impact on the way your place is set out. However, in the coming months your baby will learn to crawl. Some babies have a top speed that would impress a cheetah in hot pursuit of a wildebeest. You put them down, blink . . . and all you can see is a vapor trail of diaper fumes as they tear off down the hall.

The problem is that this new-found mobility gives your baby access to all sorts of hidden dangers around your home. Because you live your life about five to six feet or so from the floor and you hopefully have a modicum of adult intelligence, these are dangers that you would normally not have to worry about. But babies are on the ground, mobile, naturally inquisitive and have no concept of danger whatsoever.

It's really important that you baby-proof your home. Here are some ideas:

- Stairs, windows, balconies, swimming pools, fish tanks and fish ponds should be secured. Fences, railings and banisters need to have vertical slats between the bars to prevent small bodies from squeezing through or climbing over. Put gates at the head and foot of staircases to prevent unsupervised acrobatics.
- Every ground-level power outlet should be fitted with plastic plugs to prevent infant electricians from experimenting with death. Make sure that all double adapters and power strips are secure and out of reach.
- Make sure your place has electrical safety switches – technically, residual-current devices (or trip switches) – which cut the power supply in some incredible fraction of a second in the event of the baby wedging a fork into a power outlet or pulling a badly placed hair dryer into its bath. (Then again, if you are doing your job, there shouldn't be a hair dryer there anyway.) Our place is old, but it didn't cost much to get switches supplied and retro-fitted to our meter box. Baby aside, our safety switch has saved my life on three occasions. (I didn't know the toaster was plugged in.) This is an absolutely essential investment.
- All dangerous household products and objects (cleaning fluids, sprays, powders, medicines, knives, Michael Jackson DVDs, etc.) should be put in top drawers or locked cupboards. This is particularly the case in the kitchen,

bathroom and laundry. Poison control centers get 1.2 million calls every year about accidental posioning of kids under age five. A variety of easy-to-install devices is available from your local hardware store to prevent this from happening, ranging from plastic hooks to an electrified chain with a six-digit, computerized combination lock. Such a device will keep your baby out for about two or three days.

- Check that cockroach baits and mousetraps are inaccessible, and remember that kids can reach up higher than their heads. (I learned this the hard way when Rachael got her hands on a disposable razor that I'd assumed was "out of reach" and was about to clean her teeth with it.)

- Secure freestanding shelves, drawers and cupboards. Babies are good at climbing, but their King Kong-like behavior may lead to disaster if their weight is enough to topple a piece of furniture. (I wired the tops of tall and thin bookshelves to the wall to ensure there was never a book avalanche.)

- Make sure that there are no saucepan handles sticking out or power cords dangling down from anywhere. To a baby, a dangling cable is an inviting vine on which they will inevitably try to get purchase. The problem is that it is probably attached to an iron or toaster or kettle or sandwich maker. You can imagine the rest.

- Guard all fires, including heaters and stoves. If you can, keep your baby dressed in natural fibers such as cotton or wool, which are more fire-resistant than manufactured materials. Also, keep matches well away from babies. If they don't light them, they'll certainly suck them or stick them up their nose.

- Watch out for choke hazards: buttons, nuts, coins, beads, the eyes of stuffed toys and plastic bags should all be out of reach.
- Check that there are no Venetian-blind strings or curtain cords near the baby's crib or play areas. These may get tangled around its neck.
- Make sure that all things you value – especially electrical items – are suspended from the ceiling by cables or else are only accessible by ladder. Bowls of spaghetti and Blu-ray players, for example, do not coexist harmoniously.
- If your place has a low ceiling fan, be very, very careful. It's easy to forget they are up there spinning away, and when Uncle Frank comes to visit and decides to play spaceships with Baby Jessica . . . well, that's a quick end to what would otherwise have been a pleasant family gathering.

Even after you've done all these things and a couple of others that you thought up along the way, there is one more thing that you must do. It sounds a bit weird, but it's the most effective way of finding out how safe your home actually is. Here's how it works.

First, get down on your hands and knees and pretend that you are an inquisitive baby.

Second, crawl around from room to room, seeing how much damage you can do to the nice things within your reach. See if you can find some fragile ornaments to smash or precariously balanced furniture to topple.

Third, crawl around from room to room, seeing how much damage you can do to *yourself.* Find cupboards to open and things to climb on and great heights to leap off and nasty things to stick in your mouth.

Then fix all those things.

Of Cats and Dogs

Friends of mine recently had a dilemma. They had two big dogs they raised from pups who for years had been the sole guardians and masters of their house and were treated like their children. (You know the type. Their voicemail message is, "Hi. Scott, Anya, King and Snowflake can't take your call right now . . .")

This was all well and good . . . right up to the moment my friends had a *real* child, which was coincidentally the exact moment the dogs got demoted and suddenly and sadly found out where they really stood in the pecking order. Some of the canine privileges (besties sleeping at the foot of their bed) disappeared overnight. So, in a swift but ill-fated move, while mother and baby were resting in the hospital before the home-coming, my friend thought up a grand scheme to prepare the dogs for the arrival of the baby into their home.

I remember sitting in his living room the day before the big return. My friend sat his dogs down in front of him and produced from a plastic bag a wad of used diapers that he had brought from the hospital. He rubbed the dogs' faces in them while chanting the baby's name over and over: "Anna, Anna, Anna . . ."

I guess there was something deep in his frontal lobe that made sense of this. But it didn't seem quite right to me. The dogs' eyes were glistening a little too brightly for my liking. All I could think of was an old movie where a British lord threw a sweater belonging to an escaped convict to his bloodthirsty hounds. They sniffed and growled at it and then galloped off across the moors to hunt him down and rip him to pieces.

Some people are dog people. Some are cat people. Some are bird people. I'm not much of a pet person myself. I had

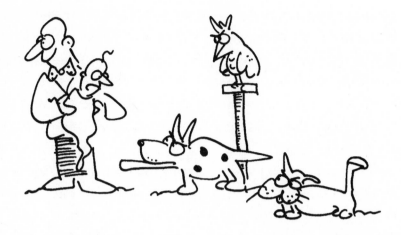

a dog when I was a kid, but I had to feed it and that meant opening tins of dog food, which scarred me for life. I vowed I'd never have a pet when I got older. I did end up getting some guinea pigs for the girls, but they were pathetic and timid creatures that died of fright in a thunderstorm. Oh, and then there was our rabbit, which escaped. I found it dead and stiff in the gutter one morning just as the girls were coming out the front door to go to school. Oh yeah, that was a day I won't forget in a hurry.

If you have a pet – dog, cat, bird, boa, turtle, whatever – you need to think through the implications of what it means to bring a new member of the family into your home. This is especially the case – be honest now – if up till this time you have treated your pet as a member of the family rather than a pet (i.e., it sleeps on your bed, climbs on furniture, licks your face). It doesn't take them long to work out that the attention once lavished on them is now directed elsewhere, and that can cause what would best be described as jealousy.

Ensure you continue to give your pet some attention to reduce its animalistic competitive streak, and, just to be safe, make sure it has no unsupervised access to your baby. Even "good" animals can give a quick nip or scratch. All light-heartedness aside, every so often there are tragedies where a family pet significantly injures or kills a child.

As far as I can make out, there are only a few pets that are safe to keep when you have a new baby in your home. Birds are stuck in a cage, so they can't fly over and attack with their steely talons. Guinea pigs, fish and mice are docile and not much of a threat . . . unless your baby tries to eat one. Turtles are aggressive, but they move so slowly that you've got about four days to head off a direct attack.

Come to think of it, ponies are probably okay too, as long as you don't let them into the nursery.

Remembering to Be a Couple

You and your wife used to be a couple. Now you're a family.

You used to be a duo. Now you're a trio (or perhaps a quadro, etc.)

You used to be tennis partners. Now you're a dodgeball team.

Here's the point. Having a baby in your home changes your relationship with your wife. This is because you don't spend as much time together as you used to. You used to go out to dinner and see bands and go for walks and watch movies and talk intimately and all those other things that couples do. You used to have lots of time to invest in the maintenance and development of your relationship.

But that was before the baby. Sure, there are lots of things you can still do, but it certainly is not as convenient anymore. The baby needs to be fed. The shopping needs to be done. The baby needs to be changed. The diapers need to be put on the line. The baby needs to be sung to sleep. The house needs a vacuum. The baby needs a bath. The dinner has to be cooked. The washing up hasn't been done in a while.

The problem is that you and your wife can end up running around doing work and baby and house-type duties and then all of a sudden wake up one morning and wonder who the strange person next to you in your bed is. The face seems oddly familiar . . . Oh, that's right . . . you're married to her!

If you're not careful, your relationship with your wife can go out the window. I've heard of parents who, after many years, when their kids leave home, sadly realize that they don't really know each other anymore. They were so busy being parents that they forgot to be husband and wife.

This is tragic.

The message is this: an essential part of being a good dad is being a good husband.

Don't neglect your wife.

You must both make a deliberate attempt to spend some time alone together – even if it is only a few desperately grabbed moments. Have a cup of coffee together, a chat about your day, a meal with just the two of you. Lie in bed talking for ten minutes before you get up. A little way down the track, you can extend this. You might be able to catch a movie or play tennis or have a swim. Talk to each other about what you are enjoying about being parents, and what things you might be struggling with.

Your relationship with your wife is really important. Don't forget it. As your child grows up, you want to be modelling to them on a daily basis what it means to have a healthy, respectful, loving relationship with each other; a relationship where you talk and have a few laughs and get some gear off your chest.

Mother's Day should not be the only day of the year your wife gets treated to something special. Mother's Day is a ridiculous concept promoted by retail outlets wanting to make a quick buck. Forget chocolates and roses. The best way to show your appreciation is by your words and actions. Give your wife love offerings such as a nice dinner or a clean bathroom floor. Watch the baby while she goes out and does whatever it is she wants to do. Tell her you love her and that you want to do that thing with the chocolate fondue and the beanbag.

Even More on Sex

Many new fathers find that sex is quickly relegated to that cobwebby part of their brain labelled "distant memory." Many parents are less interested in sex during the post-birth period.

The problem is, though, that nothing can bruise a husband's fragile machismo-ego like a wife uninterested in sex. It's easy to feel a little resentful that things aren't what they used to be. You can even resent the baby, because if it wasn't for its crying, crying, crying all the time, your sex life would be great, great, great. You can become jealous of all the attention lavished upon your baby by your wife – attention that used to be lavished upon you. Not only that, your wife's breasts seem to now be the exclusive domain of this new person in your home and you may be surprised or jealous that for you it is now "ACCESS DENIED."

In the cold light of day, however, it makes perfect sense and is very reasonable that your sex life will go through a transition period. Once you see what happens to your wife's body in childbirth, particularly if a Caesarean or episiotomy is involved, you will understand why your wife would rather be left alone for the moment, thank you very much. Let's go back to the anecdote about the umbrella and your penis. Meditate on this for a while. Imagine stretching your penis so far that you can scratch your nose with it. Imagine unmentionable acts with your scrotum and an InSinkErator. Imagine urinating a grapefruit. I'm sure you wouldn't feel like a heavy session of intense passion after that. And you wouldn't appreciate your wife giving you the "nudge-nudge, wink-wink" treatment or guilt trip either.

Her postnatal-body weight distribution and maternity bra probably don't help make her feel like Aphrodite, anyway. Rumour also has it that cracked nipples and sore or leaky breasts are not conducive to sensual arousal. If you can't comprehend this, give your pectorals a brisk rub with a sheet of sandpaper and then see how raunchy you feel.

When you start playing the role of the active dad and get into night settling and diaper changing and baby bathing, you'll get an inkling of why sex may not be an immediate priority. You are both perpetually exhausted and are lucky if you have a moment to yourselves. Sleep becomes a very valued commodity. It's also a little-known fact that newborn babies have a highly attuned psychic link with their mothers, which means they can detect any sexual arousal or activity within a 500-foot radius. This will immediately trigger a screaming response just at the "critical moment" – if you know what I mean.

In this regard, then, let your wife call the shots regarding your mutual re-entry (I'm sorry, I couldn't help it) into the world of lovemaking. You may have to explore a new route (I'm sorry again) in terms of expressing physical or sexual intimacy without it simply being "sex." Falling asleep in each other's arms turns out to be pretty satisfying.

And remember that this is a temporary stage and your sex life will return to normal. One day. Yep, those fifteen years will just fly by.

When You're Out of Your Depth

No one expects either you or your wife to be an instantaneous parental expert. Even if you have read widely, done courses and classes and spoken to parental pioneers, there will still be times when you feel out of your depth and unsure whether things are going as they should.

Your baby may not sleep well. It might look pale, or it might cough all the time. It might cry constantly without apparent reason. It might not go on the breast very well. Blotches or marks may appear on its skin.

Sometimes, you need practical advice or assistance. Other times, however, people want to give you advice even when you don't want it or need it. Suddenly, everyone is an expert and knows exactly how to solve your parental problems.

If anyone without kids of their own gives you advice, disregard it. They don't know what they're talking about. If they are persistent, ask them to change your baby's diaper. That'll shut them up. If any strangers in the supermarket try to give you advice, pretend you don't speak English.

Family is a little different. After all, your parents brought you up and you turned out okay. But remember too that it was your mom who used to put butter on your burns when you were a kid, and your dad still can't seem to put apps on his phone. My grandmother always seemed full of good ideas – but how much can I trust a woman who thinks a couple of spoonfuls of paraffin oil is a universal cure for pretty much any ailment?

Hospitals, community health centers and your doctor are good starting points for help and reassurance. In addition, there are a number of organizations that exist to help novice parents, such as:

- ZERO to THREE National Center for Infants, Toddlers, and Families;
- The Parents as Teachers program, which offers home visits and group meetings to first-time parents in some areas;
- The National Center on Fathering;
- The American Academy of Pediatrics, which offers parents advice online at healthychildren.org;

as well as many local organizations that you could find by asking friends or searching online. There is also a swathe of telephone support services that can provide advice, support and direction (Google "parent" and "helpline").

Don't hesitate in seeking advice from one of these places. Many people do it. A lot of the challenges you might encounter with your baby, such as establishing good sleeping patterns or getting baby on the breast, can be very difficult and frustrating. It might be that you need an answer over the phone, or it might be that you, mom, and baby can get help from a group class or other community resource. We had a few problems with Rachael's nocturnal crying, so Meredith sought out a center to help get into a sleep routine and found it to be excellent. Talking with trainers, health professionals, and other parents about your challenges can give you practical advice and coping mechanisms. It makes a big difference.

Don't be afraid to get help!

No Retreat, No Surrender

It's likely you've read this book because you're the kind of person who wants to be prepared for fatherhood. Good for you. I imagine you've also gone to class, looked around online, got some apps and all that. But be aware it will still be "academic" knowledge. Until you experience fatherhood in all its rewarding and painful glory, you won't really know what it's like in the 3D, quadraphonic sense. You have to *live it* to get the full sensation. Only when you feel the kick of your unborn child do you feel the thrill of expectation. Only when you see your wife give birth do you really understand how painful it is. Only when you hear crying at 3 am do you know what it is to be tired and cranky. Only when you change a diaper for the first time do you know the true meaning of nausea. Only when your baby says "I lub oo, Dabbee" when you tuck it in at night do you feel that bursting excitement and pride of fatherhood.

But that's okay.

You are not alone. Every dad who ever lived was in your shoes once too. They were as nervous and uncertain and excited as you are. And the human race seems to have got on just fine.

Sometimes, being a dad will be absolutely the best, most enjoyable, wonderful thing and everything will be clicking along nicely and you will be in the zone, just loving being a dad and a husband. But sometimes things won't go the way you plan. Being a dad is not an unbroken succession of great and wonderful times. It's not always holding hands and piggy-back rides and "I love you, Dad." There are busy times, rotten times, tired times, times when you are irritated, preoccupied and run-down. The important thing is not that you become the perfect father, because there is no such thing. The important thing is that when things don't look so good – when things go wrong, when you make mistakes – you try again, you keep going.

So, you're now (or anytime soon) the fully fledged father of a real live baby. You have navigated the pregnancy, survived the labor and stumbled through life at home with a newborn person. Soon, you will get used to this new life and you will start to feel comfortable and in control again. You will find your feet and look back and wonder what all the fuss was about in the first place.

To an extent, this is an appropriate feeling to have. But don't be deceived. Don't start relaxing. Pretty soon, your baby is going to learn to walk and talk.

Soon, your baby will turn into . . . *a toddler.*

That's when hell really breaks loose. Because if you thought living with a baby was bizarre, you ain't seen nothin' yet.

Epilogue

F inding out you're going to be a dad and then navigating the next months of pregnancy and preparing for childbirth are, no doubt about it, a big deal. The problem is that there is so much emphasis on pregnancy and childbirth that, after a while, that's all you see, as if *becoming* a dad is the end goal. You start to lose sight of the fact that *being* a dad is the important thing. Ending up with a baby in your hands is just the prologue to the story, the aperitif to the main course, the opening bars to the song, the departure gate on an overseas holiday, the . . .

While this book is coming to an end, your adventure as a dad is only just beginning.

And what an adventure it is; a life-changing adventure that, all things being equal, will continue for the rest of your life. Being the dad of a baby means you'll also end up being the dad of a toddler, a child, a teenager and, before you know it, an adult. You never stop being a dad.

When Meredith uttered those words, "I'm pregnant. We're going to be parents," all those years ago, I had no idea what that meant or what the years ahead would hold. Now I do.

If I could time travel back and have a beer with my pre-dad self, I would look sagely at him, I mean, me, and say, "Pete, it'll all be fine. Sure, the birth's a spin-out and the baby years are a bit rough going at times, but you'll survive and you are going to love being a dad. It becomes the central thing in your life. You've got the best years of your life coming up . . . seeing your kids, I mean *my* kids, well . . . okay, *our* kids – that's a bit weird isn't it? – grow up and being there to help them to guide them along the way, will give you a sense of meaning and purpose and satisfaction that I'm not sure I can even explain to you. There are play nights and birthday parties, camping trips and family holidays, days at the beach and afternoons on the sidelines, father's day breakfasts and countless hilarious and heart-warming conversations, walks in the park and flying kites. You'll teach your kids to walk, talk, use a knife and fork, read, swim, throw a ball, play musical instruments, ride a bike, drive a car and order in a nice restaurant. And one day you'll tell them goodbye at the airport and wonder where did those years go, and you'll be proud of who they are: well-balanced, well-rounded, intelligent, kind, independent, funny, loving, stylish, accomplished and gracious human beings . . . but I'm getting ahead of myself. You probably just want to focus on the birth for the moment, right? Sure. Oh, and Pete, two bits of advice before I go back to the future . . . first, that day when you go to the beach and think the swell doesn't look too bad and you decide to take your three very young children, who can barely swim, right out to it? Don't do that. And second, for your tenth wedding anniversary, don't buy Meredith a bread maker."

So to you, my paternal comrades, I offer my congratulations on being given the awesome responsibility and tremendous privilege of fatherhood. Although this might not be obvious right now, this is the biggest thing you are going to do in your life (unless you cure cancer, are the first person to walk on Mars or you invent teleportation). Embrace it in all its richness and wonder. Savor the golden times, struggle through the frustrating times, and be a good dad.

I hope in some small way this book has given you a glimpse of the joy, pain, wonder, frustration, pleasure and even comedy of dadhood. I hope it has helped you prepare for your own journey as a dad.

Becoming a dad redefined me. I used to be scared of that. Now, I am grateful. And although I never know what's coming around the next corner, I'm really, *really* looking forward to the years ahead.

I hope you are too.

Good luck on your journey . . . Dad.

Acknowledgments

The longest Oscar-award thanks took almost six minutes, and the longest movie credits roll for over twelve. Mine are considerably shorter.

Thanks to:

Meredith, my companion, wife and silent writing partner, for her love, patience and devotion to me and our children. It's easy to be a good dad when you've got a good mom by your side. It's a credit to her that she remains so loving, patient and totally devoted even after she discovered I publish lots of personal stuff about her. The places in this book where I come across as sage and learned? That is *her*.

Rachael, Georgia and Matilda, our adorable girls. I couldn't have been a dad without you. I love you and am always there for you, except when I've had a few glasses of shiraz and you want to be picked up at the bus stop on a rainy night, at which time your mother is there for you.

Hilda and Stan, my wonderful parents and role models, for always letting me know I was important.

Ray Farley, fellow author and father, for his coaching. Sue Williamson, cousin and lactation consultant, who taught me all I know about breastmilk. Dr. Stewart Montano, mate since primary school, for setting me straight about medical stuff and letting me join his Inventors' Club when we were in Third Class. Dr. Keith Hartman, obstetrician and Alfa Romeo driver, for his impressive professional skill and personal touch. Pascale Beard, for suggesting that *So You're Going to Be a Dad* is a catchier title than *Becoming a Dad: The Australian Guy's Guide to Fatherhood*. Phillip Young, who has bought more copies of this book than anyone else on the planet.

My original publishing team: Susan Morris-Yates, Executive Editor, for taking a chance with a new boy; and Stephanie Pfennigwerth, my trusty editor, who cut and slashed my ramblings into an acceptable read.

The Second Edition team: Julia Collingwood, Managing Editor, and Susan Gray, editor el-supremo for dragging me into the 21st century; and boss-man Jon Attenborough, who is just a swell guy.

And the Third Edition team: Lou Johnson, Managing Director, Larissa Edwards, Head of Publishing, Roberta Ivers, Managing Editor, and Carol Warwick, Senior Marketing and Publicity Manager, for all thinking yet another edition of this book sounded like a good idea, and eagle-eyed editor Kevin O'Brien for, well . . . editing; my friend and midwife Chloe Owens; and, back twenty years later for another round, my cousin Sue (and the Australian Breastfeeding Association), still flying the lactation flag. And, of course, Simon Schuster, publisher and all-round great guy, for inviting me to his chalet in Banff.

And a final salute to all my paternal and maternal comrades, (in particular, Mark and Ayumi Steuer, Keith and Michelle Bannister, Rusty and Michelle Terry, and Jeremy and Kathryn Martens) for reflecting upon their own experiences as new parents. Fo sho, u guys r #BFFL. Let's MySpace each other soon! ROFL!

PETER DOWNEY

Glossary

This is not an exhaustive glossary. It just contains a whole lot of words that I know relating to pregnancy, birth and parenthood.

afterbirth (i) All the stuff that comes out of the mother after the baby is born; (ii) The time immediately following the birth of the baby.

amniocentesis The extraction and testing of the amniotic fluid (see below) for abnormalities in the fetus.

amnion The inner lining of the amniotic sac, which is the bag in which the baby grows inside the mother.

amniotic fluid The fluid inside the amniotic sac, which is the bag in which the baby grows inside the mother. (When this breaks naturally and the fluid flows out, it is euphemistically referred to as "the water breaking.")

amniotic sac The bag in which the baby grows inside the mother.

amniotomy Using a hook to rupture the amniotic sac, which is the bag in which the baby grows inside the mother, releasing the amniotic fluid, which is the fluid inside the amniotic sac.

anaesthetic Helps one cope with pain, by blocking the signals to the brain. Often used by mothers during labor (injections or gas) and fathers getting used to a newborn (bourbon or beer).

antenatal Time before the birth (i.e., during pregnancy).

Apgar test A scale used immediately after birth to rate the newborn's heartbeat, breathing, skin, muscle tone, reflexes and sense of humor. Named after Dr. Virginia Apgar.

augmentation The process of making labor go faster.

baby The highly technical name given to your child after it's finished being a fetus.

Beta hCG (human chorionic gonadotropin) A nasty hormone and the harbinger of morning sickness.

bilirubin (i) The pigment that builds up in the bloodstream giving jaundiced babies their yellowish color; (ii) BTW, I went to elementary school with a kid called Billy Ruben.

birth When the baby comes out of the mother.

birth canal The passage that the baby has to navigate to get out of the mother.

blastocyst The cell structure (made up of the trophoblast and the embryoblast) that will grow into the placenta and the embryo.

blues Deep sadness experienced during postnatal period, caused by hormonal changes in the mother's body combined with massive life disruption and tiredness. Can transition into much more serious depression.

bouncer (i) A device for baby bouncing; (ii) Security employee who stands outside a bar with a piece in his ear like he works on Airforce One.

Braxton Hicks contractions Extremely inconvenient false labor contractions.

breast pump Device that looks like the bug-catcher you got for your seventh birthday. It makes *schloop, schlurp* noises and sucks breastmilk out for storage or bottling.

breech birth When the baby is born bum-first.

Caesarean section (i) The surgical removal of stubborn unborns; (ii) The Roman quarter where Caesar's supporters lived.

cervix The bottom of the uterus. Think: sump.

chromosomes Microscopic, thread-like structures that contain thousands of genes. Each cell has twenty-three chromosomes. (*See also* X chromosome and Y chromosome)

circumcision Cutting off the squidgy skin on the end of the penis. Not to be confused with castration or circumlocution.

colic A condition during which babies scream and yell and wail, and you go psycho-bananas trying to cope with it.

colostrum A rich breast secretion, jam-packed full of proteins, antibodies and other nourishing stuff, which flows for a few days after birth before the milk kicks in.

conception When the fertilized egg buries itself in the uterus.

contraceptive That horse has already bolted for you, pal.

Cook Cervical Ripening Balloon A mechanical device to encourage the opening of the cervix.

Couvade syndrome Where you are not giving birth (i.e., you are a guy) but you have symptoms that you are.

cradle cap A crusty yellow skin rash common on a newborn's scalp.

crowning The moment the baby's head appears on the way out.

delivery When somebody brings you something, such as a pizza. Or a baby.

depression An intense, serious and long-term low mood; an illness that can negatively impact all parts of life: relationships, self esteem, work, energy, physical health, sleep. It is important for mothers (or fathers) experiencing depression to seek assistance from a health professional. *See also* blues.

dilation The process of being made wider. For example, the pupils of your eyes when you enter a dark room, or the cervix when it realizes that the baby is about to try to pass through it.

embryo Another name for your child in one of its earliest stages, technically from implantation until about the twelfth week of pregnancy.

embryoblast The gathering of cells that will become a fetus and then a baby.

endorphins The body's natural opiates.

engaged When the baby gets ready for birth during the last month of pregnancy by turning into the *eject position.*

engorgement When the mother's breasts go overboard on the milk production and get bigger and bigger and sorer and sorer.

epidural The procedure of anaesthetizing the entire lower half of a woman by injecting drugs into her lower spine.

episiotomy A surgical cut in the perineum to make it bigger so the baby can get out. This is done to prevent or impede tearing.

estrogen A hormone produced in large quantities during pregnancy.

Fallopian tubes The tunnels between the ovaries and the uterus where fertilization takes place.

fertilization When the sperm and the ovum get together. This is the very first step in the production of human life.

flaccid Soft and drooping.

fetal alcohol spectrum disorder (FASD) Any of a number of different medical issues that can arise in a newborn because their mother hit the bottle during pregnancy.

fetal distress When complications arise during birth causing a shortage of oxygen to the baby; i.e., when the umbilical cord gets tangled or pinched.

fetus The name of your baby after the period when it is an embryo; technically from after the twelfth week of pregnancy until birth.

fontanelle The soft spot on the fetus's or newborn's head where the skull has yet to join together.

forceps Gigantic baby-grabbing pliers, used in difficult births.

foreskin (i) The squidgy skin covering the head of the penis; (ii) The battle cry of a soldier running towards opposing infantry, as in, "Fore-Skin and Country!"

genes Microscopically tiny things that carry genetic information within cells.

genital nub The small bud in an embryo's genital region that will develop into sexual organs. During a scan, its state can be used by a radiographer to take a good guess at the sex of the embryo.

Glands of Montgomery The bumps on a woman's nipple, named after an Irish doctor.

gynecologist A doctor specializing in a woman's reproductive system.

Hellin's Law The mathematical principle that describes one's chances of having twins, triplets, quads, etc.

hormones Chemicals in the bloodstream that act as messengers to prime specific organs in the body for some type of response. During pregnancy, women have a lot of these floating around. (Chemicals, that is, not organs.)

immunization The process whereby you protect your child from getting deadly diseases.

implantation This is when the sperm–ovum blobby thing picks out a cozy spot in the uterine wall to call home.

incubator A sealed crib used for monitoring newborns.

induction The artificial triggering of labor.

intravenous drip A slow feed line of fluid from a bag into the vein by way of a catheter.

jaundice A common newborn thing where the baby's liver doesn't process bilirubin (see above), so the baby turns yellow. If it hasn't gone away after three days, your doctor may want to check to see if there is anything else going on.

labor The hard work experienced by a woman in getting the baby out of her.

lanugo A covering of fine body hair on the developing in-utero baby which usually disappears towards the end of the pregnancy. However, some babies are born with it. Can be a bit freaky, but goes away by itself after a while.

let down (i) When a woman's milk drops into her breasts; (ii) The feeling you get when you're on a long-haul flight and you discover your entertainment unit is broken.

mastitis Painful breast problem where breasts get lumpy and as sore as testicles that have just been trodden on by Morris dancers.

meconium The technical name given to a baby's first

bowel movements. It is tacky and dangerous. Don't get it on you.

midwife A highly-trained medical practitioner who specializes in pregnancy, childbirth and mother care.

morning sickness When a woman feels gross and nauseous during pregnancy.

motility The capacity and fitness of a sperm to "swim" towards the ovum.

mucus Tacky discharge from the nose and other mucous membranes, such as the cervix.

nausea gravidarum Morning sickness.

nitrous oxide Anaesthetic also referred to as laughing gas, although I'm not sure why anyone would want to laugh during childbirth.

nuchal scan Scans the quantity of fluid within the neck of the fetus to help identify certain conditions such as Down syndrome.

obstetrician A specialist doctor and surgeon who specializes in the reproductive system.

oocyte Ovum. Egg.

operculum The all-important plug of mucus that seals the cervix, thereby allowing the baby to grow in its own sterile environment.

ova Plural of ovum.

ovary Place where ova are produced.

ovulation When the ovum comes out of the ovary.

ovum Egg from the female which when combined with a sperm creates the start of a human being. (Singular of ova.)

oxytocin A hormone that encourages uterine contraction and milk production.

pediatrician A specialist children's doctor.

pelvic floor The muscles at the base of the pelvis that hold everything together.

pelvis The bones forming the cavity in men and women's lower torsos, and also that region in general.

perineum External skin all around the vagina and anus.

pethidine A type of anaesthetic delivered by injection.

placenta The interface between mother and fetus that controls life-support and waste disposal.

placentophagy The act of eating the placenta, post birth.

posterior In relation to childbirth, this is when the baby is head-first in the birth canal but on its back rather than on its front. Although babies can be delivered in this way, the preferred birth position is head-first and on its front.

postnatal Time after the birth.

postpartum depression *See* depression.

premature When a baby is born before the 37th week of pregnancy, meaning that its organs may not be fully developed enough to cope with independent survival. A premature baby requires specialist care.

prenatal *See antenatal.*

progesterone A hormone produced in large quantities during pregnancy.

prostaglandin A hormone that encourages labor contractions. It is found in prostaglandin gel, pessaries and semen.

rooting reflex When a baby pokes around on the breast looking for the nipple.

scrotum Wrinkly, dangly male sac containing the all-important testicles.

semen The goopy stuff, containing sperm, that comes out of your penis during orgasm.

show A sign of the onset of labor, when the cervical plug that has been sealing the mother's cervix detaches and comes out via the vagina.

SIDS Sudden infant death syndrome. The sudden, unexpected and inexplicable death of a baby under one year of age, that occurs during sleep.

sperm The male reproductive tadpole. There are about 300 million sperm per human ejaculation, which, though impressive, is not as awesome as that of the pig, which produces about forty-five billion a go. That's billion, not million. The hamster, on the other hand, has only a fairly uninspiring 3000, which is why there are so few hamsters around.

stirrups A device integral to the Universal Television Birthing Position, used to hold a laboring mother's legs akimbo during birth; Also used by equestrians to hold their feet up while riding.

stitches When you get sewn up; usually applicable to the perineum.

Syntocinon A synthetic hormone that helps contract the uterus.

TENS machine A medical device that provides transcutaneous electrical nerve stimulation (experienced as pulses) through pads placed on the skin. Used in physical therapy and pain relief situations.

term The period of the pregnancy. To go to full term is to carry the baby to the end of the pregnancy.

testicles You should have two of these unless you played soccer when you were a kid, in which case one might be wedged back up where it's not supposed to be. This is the storage tank for your sperm; also referred to as the family jewels, goolies or squids.

transition The painful period between the first and second stages of labor.

trimester A third of the full term of pregnancy; i.e., three months.

trophoblast The cell structure that forms the beginnings of the placenta. Part of the blastocyst.

ultrasound The technological wonder that creates a picture of the fetus by using high-frequency soundwaves. It's like a sonar but, instead of looking for enemy submarines, you're looking for hands, feet and a head.

umbilical cord The supply line between the mother and the fetus.

UTBP The Universal Television Birth Position, which is with mother on her back and her legs up in stirrups.

uterus Place where the baby grows; also known as the womb.

vagina Yeah, like you need a definition for this?

ventouse Baby-removing device that uses vacuum sucking to lock onto baby and assist its transition out of the mother.

vernix The creamy goop used by newborn babies for lubrication on its way down the birth canal and to keep warm when it finally gets out.

water Euphemism for the fluid inside the amniotic sac. When the water "breaks," all the fluid pours out onto the floor, or the expensive lounge suite, or wherever the woman happens to be at the time.

wind Babies have lots of this. It means they have air in their stomachs and it has to come out via the holes at both ends of their bodies.

womb (i) Another word for uterus; (ii) The airy sound produced when a boomerang whistles past your ears: *womb womb womb womb womb.*

X chromosome A genetic sex indicator. All ova are X. If an X sperm fertilizes the ovum, the baby will be a girl.

Y chromosome A genetic sex indicator. If a Y sperm fertilizes the ovum, the baby will be a boy.

You bastard Term of endearment directed at a husband by his wife in the throes of labor.

Zygote The cell formed by the combination of ovum and sperm, that will grow in time into an embryo, fetus, baby, child and high school graduate.

Zzzzz What you don't get enough of as father of a baby.

Appendix I

Parental Education Films

A lot of guys learn from movies and TV series, and there are plenty of them that deal with – or at the very least contain informative scenes about – conception, pregnancy, labor and life at home with a new baby. Some are better than others. Here are my suggestions of the ones to see . . . and the ones to avoid. These are just my opinions, of course, but my opinions are very, very good.

Alien
Watch, and be grateful that human babies aren't born like this.

Alien Resurrection
The alien has a baby. Again, be grateful that human babies aren't born like this.

Babies (1990)
Hollywood slop. Young couples struggle through pregnancy, sperm testing, infertility, ultrasounds and so on, and all is wholesome at the end. Amazing labor sequence as mother gives birth to a clean eight-month-old!

Babies (2010)
An oddly delightful, subtle and hugely acclaimed documentary tracking four babies – Bayar, Mari, Hattie and Ponijao – during their first year of life. Makes you realize there is more than one way to raise a child.

Baby Boom
No, not a film about a dynamite truck crashing into a maternity ward. Instead, Diane Keaton is a successful businesswoman and a competent, full-time mother.

Baby of the Bride
What do American soap stars do in their off season? Make saccharine drivel like this, where hordes of them flaunt the clichés of pregnancy and childbirth.

Baby Talk
Yuppie couple strive for pregnancy. Clichés everywhere. See the special-effects wizardry as mother gives birth to a baby with a navel!

The Back Up Plan
Some cultures around the world might consider America a vacuous, inane and unworthy place. This film has contributed to that sentiment.

Big Daddy
Adam Sandler teaches his infant son to urinate in public. Against a wall, I think.

The Brady Bunch Christmas Special
Contains the most unrealistic labor sequence ever filmed.

Call the Midwife
A popular BBC series tracking the adventures of a group of midwives in post-WWII London.

Carrie (2013)
A horrendous solo home birth in which Julianne Moore gives birth to a clean baby with no umbilical cord. Amazing!

The Color Purple
Contains a fairly realistic birth sequence. As a bonus, see Oprah before she was famous.

Dances with Wolves: The Director's Cut
A very long film, good for those long nights with a screamer.

Dirty Dancing
A delightful film with an engaging eighties soundtrack all about how it is not right to put a baby in a corner. Whatever that means.

Don't Tell Mom the Babysitter's Dead
Not to be watched before your first babysitting experience.

Everything You Wanted to Know About Sex, but Were Afraid to Ask
See Woody Allen play a sperm about to meet his fate.

The Exorcist
This is a good film to prepare you for labor.

The Fast and the Furious 6
Sure, on one level this film could be seen as plotless nonsense made up of ludicrous stunts, cheesy one-liners, comedically huge tattooed biceps, mindless violence, offensive sexual and racial stereotypes, car porn, invincible villains, clichéd dialogue, inane techno-babble, pretty explosions, incomprehensible jumps in narrative logic, old-school "I have many computer screens therefore I can hack anything within ten seconds" type techno guff, the throaty gravitas of Vin Diesel and an airport runway in the explosive grand finale that must be easily over thirty-five miles long . . . but you have to look beyond that to the touching subtext of a guy (Paul Walker RIP) just working out what it means to be a dad. Birth scene at 01:58 and then his awesome dad skills in the movie's closing moments? I cried.

For Keeps
Real footage of conception over the credits. Molly Ringwald and her husband try to balance diapers, postpartum depression, work and parenting while their lives fall apart. The birth sequence is quite realistic and even has a real newborn playing the part of the real newborn. Ignore the sequence where mom holds the baby in her lap in the car.

The Hand that Rocks the Cradle
Another "not to be watched before your first babysitting experience" film.

Juno
Teenage girl gets pregnant and is kind of together about the whole deal. Critical acclaim . . . but I thought it was a bit odd.

Knocked Up
I inexplicably like this unbelievable film, maybe because I related to the main character, a dope who ends up being an unplanned dad. (Or it could be because it stars Katherine Heigl? Yes, I think so.) One of Judd Apatow's early and better films.

Life As We Know It
Color by numbers rom-com about two gorgeous things who inherit their friends' baby and find love in the blah blah . . . I think it's a terrible film, but Katherine Heigl is in it, and that has to count for something.

Look Who's Talking
Great special-effects sequence over the credits of sperm hunting for the ovum followed by the development of the fetus.

Made in America
Worth seeing just for the quirky sperm-donation sequence. After that, switch it off.

Maybe Baby
Very British comedy from Ben Elton. Joely Richardson struggles to get pregnant.

Meet the Fockers
Fluffy comedy with a bizarre scene where Robert De Niro shows his invention that allows men to "breastfeed" using a

fake-breast harness. This scene was filmed by professionals under controlled conditions and should not be attempted at home.

Mr. Mom
Michael Keaton plays a full-time dad and finds that it is not as easy as it looks.

Nine Months
Hugh Grant and Julianne Moore become unplanned parents.

One Born Every Minute
Popular "fly on the wall" documentary series (both in UK and US versions) tracking the birth experiences of couples from all walks of life. Compulsive viewing, but be warned: pretty graphic.

Parenthood
Steve Martin shows what lies ahead for us dads. Great stuff despite the clichéd scene of cigar smoking in the waiting room.

Robin Williams Live
Stage show including some comical insights into labor and parenting.

Rosemary's Baby
Woman gives birth to the Antichrist. Don't let your wife see it.

She's Having a Baby
One of the best fatherhood education films ever made. Naive Father Type I faces the trials of sperm testing, birth classes

and the hospital experience. Realistic labor sequence and excellent suggestions for baby names over the final credits.

Spawn
Woman gives birth to hideous alien. Don't let your wife see this one either.

Star Wars: Revenge of the Sith
Labor sequence of Luke and Leia being born. Then mother dies.

Three Men and a Baby
One of the best fatherhood education films ever made. Three successful corporate guys (Danson, Guttenberg and Selleck) are thrown headlong into "fatherhood." Great insights into feeding, diapers, bathing and shopping.

Trois Hommes et un Couffin
The original *Three Men and a Baby*, but in French.

The Walking Dead, Season 3, Episode 4
Worst C-Section ever. Mom gets one with her son's pocket knife in a prison cell while zombies roam outside. If your wife has a Caesarean, it will be heaps better than this.

What to Expect When You're Expecting
I'll tell you exactly what to expect . . . Not much beyond cardboard characters, clichéd conversations and yet another movie suggesting the only way to give birth is with your feet up in stirrups.

Appendix II

What My Friends Had to Say

Since the vibe of this book is "the common man's experience" of fatherhood, I invited some of my fathering comrades to have their say as well. I asked them to free-associate about pregnancy, birth, life as a dad and whatever else came to mind (thereby ensuring they will buy their own copy of the book, instead of borrowing mine).

So, here it is – the wisdom of those who have walked the road ahead of you. Read it with a grain of salt.

Adrian
father of Lyndall, six weeks

From the age of fifteen, I planned out my life . . . what sort of job I would like, the type of girl I wanted to marry, and the place where I wanted to live. I fulfilled my plans but with a pregnant wife found myself feeling uncomfortably out of control.

The first part of the pregnancy was really rough, with a threatened miscarriage. I was quite anxious about being at the birth, but I was trusting in someone greater than me. I was praying everything would be okay.

When the day came, Annie's water broke at home so we scrambled to the hospital. It was really exciting. When we arrived, she was two centimeters dilated. I put on my swimsuit and got in the shower with her. Then things got wild. It all happened so fast, I was in shock. The pains came hard and sharp. I didn't know what was going on. Thirty minutes later, Lyndall was born. I was overwhelmed. Two hours later, I was still gaga. I was totally occupied with my new family. That was when the doctor pointed out that I was still in my swimsuit and I should probably put some clothes on.

Al

father of Amy, nine, Beth, seven, Gareth, five, and Josephine, two
My advice? Be around and make it fun to be a kid.

Andrew

father of Zoe, eight weeks
Everyone kept telling me that being a dad was going to really change things. I haven't found it to be like that at all. I expected my life to be over. Some things of course have changed, but it's nothing you can't adjust to.

We've just come back from four weeks' hiking and camping, with Zoe bobbing around in a front sling. She survived four-wheel-driving and a jog down Kosciuszko to escape a storm. Our tent even collapsed one night and she didn't even wake up. On one part of the trip, Gaia kayaked while I drove the car with the baby in it down a riverside road. When she needed a feed, I'd just pull over and honk the horn.

I think it's all a matter of attitude. If you focus on the negative and talk yourself into a corner, you'll of course end up being defeatist and looking for problems in the whole thing.

In terms of the birth itself, that was pretty wild. I came home from work and Gaia had walked a few kilometers up to the hospital. I got up there about four in the afternoon and we went through till seven the next morning. We were even sleeping in three-minute bursts between contractions – we were so exhausted.

When Zoe was born, I was just blown away. It was the most awesome thing to see. I've done lots of stuff in my life [at] the four ends of the globe, but the birth was the most amazing thing I've ever encountered.

Bill

father of Talitha, three days

Everyone keeps telling me that BC stands for Before Children. It makes me nervous and curious as to the changes in our life-style. I am hoping and praying that I can meet the challenges and be a good father.

The birth was pretty moving. We went to the hospital and then got sent home again because nothing was happening. By the time we got home, the contractions had started again. We went back to the hospital. That was at 4 pm. Talitha was born around four the next morning. I was surprised that I was invited to "catch" her on the way out. She was so slimy! I'm glad it wasn't me giving birth.

David

father of Simon, three, and Timothy, fifteen months

As a father, you don't have to be one of *The Magnificent Seven* . . . but here's the Good, the Bad and the Ugly of being a father.

The Good: that magic moment when the head first crowns, the first smiles, first steps, first words and cuddles.

The Bad: sleep deprivation, sleep deprivation and sleep deprivation.

The Ugly: ties stained with breastmilk vomit, first solids, leaking diapers.

Eric

father of twins Harrison and Jordan, eight months

I don't think you can imagine how hard it'll be. I've got seven nieces and nephews, some of whom I helped raise. But holding down a job and living with them twenty-four hours a day under the one roof . . . that's another story.

It's fifty times harder and a hundred times better than I ever imagined. My advice? Get all the help you can.

Gabi

father of Daniel, ten, and Joel, seven

My first thought when I got into the labor room was, "There's no way that baby is gonna fit through there!" The labor was pretty exhausting. What I remember most is the hunger I felt. Deb went into labor at midnight and twenty hours later I still hadn't eaten. We got all psyched up for a natural childbirth and then they realized the baby was posterior and [had] got into distress, so Deb had to go off for a Caesarean. That was a bit unexpected. And, to be honest, there came a fear that something might go wrong.

When we brought the baby home, it didn't change our lives much. We still made it to restaurants and just put him under the table! The big change was that I used to be a surfer. Gone were the days of getting my board and heading out for an afternoon of waves. Taking a baby to the beach meant umbrellas and bassinets, clothes . . . oh, you name it. The surfing had to go.

Grant

father of Alex, three, and William, three days

Becoming a father is full of unexpected joys and spontaneous pleasures. Children make life simpler but richer. They bring less peace but greater fulfillment. Accept all the advice you can handle, ask for help when you need it and don't overlook your wife.

James

father of Anna, six hours

The prenatal classes turned out to be a waste of time because we didn't do any of the stuff we'd practiced. My wife didn't want to be walked or rocked or massaged.

It was frustrating when all the staff were saying, "Look, there's the head," and stuff like that. I couldn't see a thing because she had me in a headlock. I felt like I was in a rugby scrum. I was really surprised when Anna was born. She was covered in a thick white cream, like glue. Anyway, it was bloody exciting. Unbelievably emotional. I wouldn't have missed it for anything.

Jamie

superfather of twins Caleb and Daniel, two, and twins Sam and Hannah, eight months

When Annie started showing at five weeks, everyone started getting suspicious. She grew rapidly. When she had the ultrasound, it confirmed that we were having twins. We were really excited. My only fear was that there were more than two in there.

But the second time was different. I never, never thought for one moment that we would have twins again . . . I thought that it was statistically unlikely and I kept telling myself not to worry.

When I found out, I was in a state of shock. Four kids in two and a half years . . . I didn't know anybody who had lived through it. The next morning, though, I was fine.

It's such a fantastic moment when your child is born. You hold him up and look into his face for a moment and it's almost like you're holding a mirror. It's such a buzz when the nurses exclaim, "Doesn't he look like his dad!" To see yourself recreated like this is breathtaking, and it's something that makes being a dad so special.

For me, seeing myself in my kids and sharing so many experiences together, watching them grow and [having] the privilege of looking after them is what makes being a dad important. Having four kids in the house . . . it's hard, but it's not overwhelming. Our babies have been really good, and it's pretty special holding a baby or two in each arm. It makes you feel . . . tall.

Jeffrey

father of Nathaniel, four, Tyler, two, and The Bump, T minus seven months and counting, foster father of Dugald, thirty-four, and Tyrone W. Dawg, four

They say that nothing can prepare you for being a father. Well, babies don't come with a set of instructions like my software, but I actually think that everything in life prepares you for being a father.

Like, for example, gridiron. You have your first child and it's two on one. That's pretty easy. You have your second and it's one on one. That's still manageable. After that, you get into zone defense plays. The kids know all the moves. Each parent marks one child each, but that still leaves one to wreak havoc. They work it all out beforehand.

Or science. Each kid is like a charged nuclear particle. Their behavior is dependent on how much space they have to move in, the ambient temperature, how fast they're travelling, how many collisions they have and how many other particles there are in the immediate vicinity. Then you introduce control rods: the parents. They absorb all the energy and prevent huge amounts of destruction occurring.

Having a new baby in the house does change things. You miss the little spur-of-the-moment things, even like getting on your bikes and going for a ride. It's physically tiring, but not really exhausting. I mean, it's not too different than studying to get through school or staying out a lot. But it takes a truckload of mental energy. Babies demand your attention all the time. You can't just leave them to amuse themselves. (My favorite age is four to seven months, which is when they're at what I call the Self-Entertaining-Non-Mobile stage. You can put a rattle in their hand in their crib and get to the fridge or bathroom for five minutes and you know they'll be where you left them when you get back.)

Being a dad is rewarding and humbling. It's helped me appreciate my own parents and put it all into perspective. You take your own parents for granted, but when you have kids you realize how much time and effort it takes. It's an incredible responsibility molding a person. Scary, but exciting.

Jeremy
father of male fetus, T minus seven weeks and counting
My wife feels all clucky and gooey and, to be honest, I sometimes stare at the little moving blob on the scan monitor and feel nothing. At times, I have imagined holding our child in my arms, as a way to elicit some sort of chemical reaction in the brain. I suspect that all my hibernating mushy feelings will proudly display themselves once we have a successful landing.

Somehow, I haven't minded all the emotional outbursts, and the constant updates on the kicking, and all the "unable to help around the house." Perhaps my lot as a father is an extraordinary gift of patience while this pregnancy is going on.

I've been to all-day seminars on breastfeeding, and been told and told and told that there will be sleepless nights, and that I won't be able to let the little tyke out of my sight (especially once he's a crawler), and that "no, we don't have everything we need" despite the accumulation of baby-paraphernalia in his room. I think I feel "told out."

In many ways, the preparation has felt draining, even the little bit that I've been involved with, and I can't really imagine either the joy or the challenges to come. But I'm looking forward to it . . .

Jim

father of Michelle, three, and Madeleine, seven months

Everyone has heard stories about new fathers and how nothing can really prepare you for it. It makes you appreciate your own parents as you never thought you would. It makes you realize your own selfishness and it gives you a new sense of responsibility.

The birthing process is extremely stressful, mainly because you feel helpless. At the same time, the imminence of the birth itself is really exciting.

I remember a great relief when our baby was born. The pain for my wife was over and our baby had all the right bits and pieces. It is not an experience a woman should go through alone. My baby looked lovely . . . not like those ordinary ones that other people have.

Nowadays, my life has totally changed. No longer do I have all the time to self-indulge the way I used to. There's no doubt I sometimes wish I could get more done, but the time with your kids is worth too much.

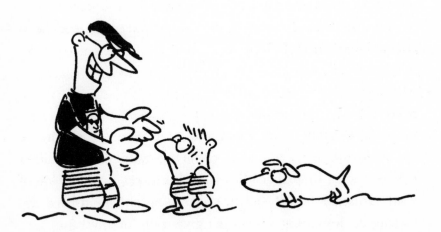

John
father of Angus, nineteen months

A hood is a garment. But there are no similarities between the state in which I find myself and any garment I have ever worn. Clothing is easily donned and removed at the whim of the wearer. Not so with fatherhood. It is not something into which one slips casually. Once acquired, it is something so integral to one's being that it can never be removed. Fatherhood affects every aspect of one's life: daily routines, sleeping habits, social life, finances – nothing escapes the influence of that bundle of joy.

All the information and advice in the world (no doubt all contained in Downey's weighty tome!) cannot prepare one for the extremes of emotion at the birth, the mind-numbing exhaustion as one sets off for work after a week of sleepless nights spent having one's ears assaulted by the screams of a baby for whom one doesn't know what to do, and the myriad other experiences that await one on the other side.

So what does fatherhood have to recommend it? Nothing can prepare you for what is in store when that little face lights up with a smile. The pleasure of fatherhood is so deep and so lasting that it easily surpasses the short-lived pleasure experienced during the baby's creation.

John
father of David, five months

I always thought that, when the time came, I would be Superdad and that it would all come naturally to me. It didn't take me long to realize that fathering takes a whole lot of work, frustration, self-sacrifice and humility. It's turned my life upside down, but I wouldn't give it up for anything.

I've done lots of things in my life that have given me satisfaction and a buzz. Being a dad, however, has been better. It's given me a sense of completeness as a person.

Kevin

father of Callaghan, two, and fetus, T minus four months and counting
Our second baby is due in four months' time and I'm dreading the labor (while hastily acknowledging that it is, of course, immeasurably harder for the woman). I don't think I acquitted myself too well the first time around, even though I was giving it my all. I kept saying things to show my compassion and support, such as "Is this helping?," "How was that position for you?," "Was that a bad one?," "Should we get your dilation measured again?" until my wife finally bellowed at me, "Stop asking me bloody questions!"

But the actual moment of birth – the crowning, followed by the unfeasibly large arm being pulled out elbow first, and then by the truly astonishing sight of Callaghan being delivered in all his large, perfectly formed, abstract-no-longer glory – was incredible.

And now, at any time of the day when I'm apart from my son – working, travelling, drifting off to sleep at night – I just have to think of him to feel a rush of happiness and wellbeing. The idea of that being doubled is fantastic.

Malcolm

father of Rebecca, two, and Joshua, seven months
Let me warn you. To go anywhere with kids involves a car-load of strollers, cribs, highchairs, changes of cool clothes, changes of warm clothes, sunhats, toys and books. You're going to

need a bigger car. Suddenly, your house doesn't seem so big or so clean.

To go anywhere without your kids involves cajoling, persuading and begging friends, family or babysitters. You find yourself staying home a lot.

And I didn't used to consider 6:30 am a sleep-in, either. But nothing prepared me for my daughter's declaration of, "I love you, Daddy," or the beaming grin that erupts over the face of my son when I walk through the door at night.

Mark
father of Hugo, six months

The Dad from Snowy River
There was movement in the belly, and a grimace on the face
For constipated was the little babe
He had started eating solids, consumed a thousand grams
And all the experts gathered at the fray.
All the tried and noted midwives from centers near and far
Had mustered at the homestead overnight
For midwives love hard feces and the challenges it brings
And Grandma snuffs the battle with delight.

There were other mothers there, from the local mothers' group
Who'd come along to lend the mom a hand
Their ideas were so varied, all had something to say
And all were quick to praise the latest brand.
As Dad lurked in the background, he looked a little tense,
So no one turned to him for his advice
But he'd been to all the courses, he'd followed all the blogs
So You're Going to Be a Dad he had read thrice.

The pain was getting stronger, the poor babe's face went red
The groaning and the moans went up a tone
The mother too was anxious, for nothing seemed to work,
Then part of a great turd did start to show.
So Dad rolled up his sleeves, approached the little babe,
And pinched the poo between finger and thumb
He pulled out the offender, and all sighed a great relief
The father–child bond had just begun.

Mark

father of Laura, three, and Katie, twenty-one months

Fatherhood . . . ah, who wouldn't want to be a father? It's wrecked my life but who's counting? It's great. Wonderful stuff. No, really. I have the best kids in the world. I enjoy being their dad. I love the smell of diapers in the morning.

Matthew

father of Jordan, one week

Look, I'm not particularly fazed about it all. It's been done a million times before. And if everybody else on the planet can do it, we can too.

I don't want our lives to be dictated by the baby. If we go out to dinner, we'll put the baby in its car seat and take it with us. Maybe I'm naive. I don't know. I mean, I know we'll spend more time at home, but I don't want to get locked away like in a fortress or something.

We've been stashing money so Tracey can take time off work, and then I'll take my leave and we'll swap the care-taking. That'll give me about three months solid at home. What a great opportunity!

Owen

father of Sophie, two, and Rosanna, two months

The worst thing I could imagine about having a baby was not getting enough sleep. So, to prepare ourselves for the worst, we fully expected what is referred to in baby-rearing circles as "a screamer." I'm not sure if it's possible to store up sleep for a later date, but I calculated that, by the time Sophie arrived, we could have gone without a decent sleep-in for about six months.

Strangely, our new arrival had no trouble sleeping through the night, sometimes for more than twelve hours straight. We kept tiptoeing into her room to hold a mirror up to her nose to see if she was still breathing. I think we learned that trick off *Murder She Wrote.*

When Rosie came along, I suspected it might not be too much more work. It's more like tag-team parenting now. One stops; the other one starts. The babies seem to know. In a way, it's twice the work, but it's certainly twice the fun.

Phil

father of Samuel, five, Laura, three, and Cameron, six weeks

The births have been the most amazing experiences. Just being there has been incredible. We went to a birth center, where the father plays an important role. I was helping with hot packs, massages, showers, gentle rocking . . . you know, just being there.

When each of my kids was born, I bawled my eyes out. It's just so miraculous and exciting. You finally see and hold your new baby.

I think it's gotten easier the more kids we've had. The first was a bit of a shock to our domestic sphere but then all the baby stuff – crying, diapers, interrupted sleep – became the norm. I've found the third one really easy. I love being a family man and watching my kids grow up.

Ray

father of Lachlan, two

Parenthood messes up your life – *Ray.*

No it doesn't – *Ray's wife.*

Actually, it's parents who mess up your life – *Ray's son.*

Mind you, I could have done without the competition – *Ray's cat.*

My life is now complete – *Ray's mother-in-law.*

It's the only worthwhile thing he's ever done in his life – *Ray's mother.*

No comment – *Ray's father.*

He should spend more time on his golf swing – *Ray's father-in-law.*

Seriously, before my wife and I stopped using contraception, we asked a few friends what it was like to be parents. The thing they emphasized was that unless you really, really, really, really, really, really want children, you shouldn't have them. This was an understatement.

So, if you're about to be a father, I'll tell you this: Every fear you have is worse than you expect, and every hope is better.

Rusty

father of Samantha, five months

When we found out M was pregnant, we were primarily concerned about how a kid would put a dampener on our social lives, and as it turned out . . . it did. Massively . . . and quite in the way we had imagined. We do have far less time to spend on our own interests, but now I really enjoy spending this time with my family!

While there was a lot to get used to straight off the bat (i.e., why is this thing still crying?), I have to say I have found real joy in just the little things I experience with our daughter.

My dad told me that he never changed more than four diapers in his life . . . And he had four kids! I don't know how he got away with it. I regularly change more than four diapers in a day, and considering the variety of interesting surprises that my daughter leaves for me I sometimes wish things hadn't changed that much. (We haven't even started her on solids yet . . .) Saying that, I really do value and enjoy being involved in the day to day caring of Samantha.

Sandy
father of The Unborn, T minus six months and counting
Pascale brought home a pregnancy kit just to stir me. She'd just come off the pill, so it was a bit of a joke.

The smile was wiped off our faces when the little strip turned purple. We just sat there and stared at it, waiting for it to fade. It didn't.

The next morning, she got up and checked it. Still purple. In fact, it's been several weeks now, it's still purple. We check it every morning. Every morning, it's still purple.

It's slowly starting to dawn on us what this little purple strip means . . . It's hard to come to terms with. It just . . . "happened." The funny thing is, I don't feel like I'm a "parent." I'm just a normal guy.

Simon
just married
Look, Pete, I know I'm not a dad yet but I'm trying really hard, honest! Give us a few years and we'll be right into this parenting thing. Can't I be in your book, please?

Simon

father of Christina, six months

One of the best things about being a dad is crashing out in the lounge room on a Sunday afternoon with my daughter and enjoying the rugby together. She is such an enthusiastic spectator: eyes wide, arms flapping and legs kicking. She doesn't care who wins, as long as they wear a red sweater.

Just by being there, my daughter turns an ordinary event into a special one. What does concern me, however, is how she is in the habit of calling out "Daddadadda" to every player on the field.

Wayne

father of Brittainy, eighteen months

Look, Pete, I was going to try to have it ready by tonight but I'm too damn busy being a father. Hey . . . why don't you just print that?

Index